Ethical Challenges Involved in the Treatment and Control of HIV AIDS An Analytical Study in Medical Ethics

Surya Rao

CONTENTS

	Page No.
CHAPTER – I	
INTRODUCTION	1-19
CHAPTER – II	
ETHICAL THEORIES AND PRINCIPLES RELEVANT TO MEDICAL PROFESSION	20-52
CHAPTER – III	
ETHICAL ISSUES INVOLVED IN HIV/AIDS SCREENING	53-81
CHAPTER – IV	
LEGAL AND MORAL ISSUES RELATING TO AIDS	82-119
CHAPTER – V	
AIDS CARE PHYSICIANS AND SOCIETY PERCEPTION	120-149
CHAPTER – VI	
AIDS STIGMA AND DISCRIMINATION: ETHICAL CONFRONTATIONS	150-201
CHAPTER – VII	
ETHICAL ISSUES CONCERNED WITH AIDS DRUGS, VACCINE TRIALS AND INSURANCE	202-249
CHAPTER – VIII	
CONCLUSION	250-298
BIBLIOGRAPHY	299-324
ARTICLES PUBLISHED IN NATIONAL AND INTERNATIONAL JOURNALS	325-330

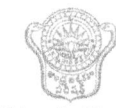

Andhra University, Visakhapatnam

Chapter

One

Introduction

Andhra University, Visakhapatnam

CHAPTER – I

INTRODUCTION

Ever since the dawn of human civilization, the personal as well as social behaviour of human beings has been controlled and regulated by a set of moral rules and conventions. Apart from the common rules and standards of human behaviour, there is a special code of conduct prescribed to the individuals of every profession. Whatever profession a person chooses to work, it is obligatory to him to follow the rules prescribed for that profession.

Human life is basically value-oriented. To make human life worth living, it must be based on certain morals and values. Medical ethics or health care ethics is concerned with the values appropriate to the professionals working in the field of medical practice. It deals with physician-patient relationship, the principles of beneficence and nonmaleficence, dedication to profession, duties to patients, confidentiality and truth telling, respect for individual dignity and autonomy, freedom of choice and informed consent etc. Sometimes conflict of interest may arise in these areas, and medical profession seeks to codify a set of rules to guide their members.

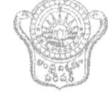

Medical treatment for curing certain human diseases is not like repairing some defective parts of a machine. It deals with human persons, and as such, it goes beyond the techniques used in a machine to human problems. Curing a disease means restoring the person to his normal health for performing his routine functions or duties. Curing a disease is a teamwork, which includes the doctor, the nurse, and the allied professionals, and at times, specialists belonging to other branches of medicine such as neurology, nephrology, cardiology and gastroenterology etc. Every person involved in the treatment of the patient supports each other and takes responsibility in curing the disease.

As a physician practicing medicine for the last two and half decades, and as a specialist in the care and treatment of HIV / AIDS, I had an opportunity, to attend about 115 national and international conferences, and presented research papers on HIV/AIDS besides publishing several papers in the national and international journals. In the course of my research and investigations, I have come across certain ethical issues related to treatment of HIV/AIDS, and it has motivated me to choose the present topic, and to undertake an analytical study of medical ethics in relation to AIDS.

Since the discovery of HIV a quarter century ago[1], the scientific research has led to remarkable discoveries in this area. Today, individuals living with HIV can expect to live a relatively normal lifespan if they are diagnosed and treated in the early stages of the infection, and they are able to access and adhere to potent antiretroviral drug regimens. Thus, a deadly disease like AIDS, has been transformed into a chronic manageable condition, largely due to the efforts and research carried on by the scientists. But the spread of HIV is continuing irrespective of the difference between rural and urban areas.

At this juncture, the migration plays an important role in the geographic spread of HIV all through the country, and it is commonly found in urban centers and along highway transport routes. Women constitute one half of India's population. Yet the ground reality is still harsh for them. Rapid urbanization and migration of rural population to urban pockets in search of livelihood, has moved the epidemic through its heterosexual route inviting migrant men to indulge in high risk behaviour with sex workers. Trapped in the vicious cycle of poverty and lack of awareness, they act as a 'bridge population,' in turn infecting their partners. Women are more vulnerable to HIV infection. Only 54 percent of women are literate as compared to 76 percent of men. At least 4.5 million girls are out of primary schools, which is double the number of boys. According to the World Bank estimates, for every 1,00,000 children born, 450 women die while giving birth. Women are also vulnerable due to lack of awareness on the modes of HIV transmission, preventive measures, and low use of condoms by men. Most women are unable to negotiate safe sex or demand basic health services.[2]

Added to this is the haunting stigma attached to AIDS, and it is killing people mercilessly whether they are young or old. The twenty moral values in respect of caring for AIDS patients is a day to day predicament.

As a physician, I honestly consider, respect for human life is the primary moral duty of every medical professional. This principle, that is, respect for human life is included in the Geneva Declaration of the World Medical Association.[4] Respect for human life is a moral assertion. This does not, however, mean preserving life at all costs.

Medicine is an applied science and the principles of medical ethics are maxims that come into being from human experiences and case studies. From the time of Hypocrites, the profession of medicine has been based on both science and ethics. Medicine is not just descriptive but it's also prescriptive. Hippocrates' philosophy of "patient-doctor relationship", emphasizes maintaining 'confidentiality', and showing concern to save the life of a patient at any cost, is valid even today in respect of HIV/AIDS patients. Hypocrites' oath dictates moral obligations of doctors in providing medical services to their patients. While dealing sensitive patients both Darwinian evolution of nature on the one hand and cultural evolution on the other are important because they place limitations on each other.[5]

What is Medical Profession and How is it Related to Ethics?

Medical profession is a holistic approach for the overall wellbeing of a patient. It is an art and a science, to be more specific, 'art of skills' and 'application of medical science'. It is a patient centered, and team based discipline, directing towards a solution for health problem. By definition, the medical practice has many components such as, history taking, arriving at a provisional diagnosis, and intervention planning. It includes consideration of the subjective elements of the patients, their individual history, past history, health beliefs, life expectations and goals, and the cultural and socio-economic factors. In the era of consumer courts and expensive laboratory tests, the financial background of individual patients is to be critically measured by treating doctors, well before they suggest suitable therapeutic measures. Medical practice is not related to the world of fantasy, but it is a complex phenomenon involving doctors, patients, diseases, and drugs interacting with each other at the practical level. Hence, people engaged in medical practice should maintain a balance between doctor-patient relation, disease and drugs, following certain ethical values for it's glorification.

Medicine is a science, but practicing medicine is an art. Thus, medical practice is both an art and a science, and it should maintain equilibrium between these two.

The professional life of a Medical Practitioner is varied and dependant upon a high level of communication skills and clinical challenges. Social and psychological factors weigh heavily in the diagnostic approach of a doctor or a general practitioner (GP). The GP helps patients with early symptoms of illness as well as those with chronic illness, and GPs must be skilled in the long term management of a large variety of physical and psychiatric problems. No other specialty offers such a wide array of treating everything from pregnant women to babies and from mental illness to sports medicine.

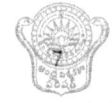

General practitioner (GP) is a front line soldier in the battle against disease. He is the first person to face the patient, and there's nothing more challenging to him than the first encounter with the patient. Normally a specialist sees the patient at a secondary level, and a super specialist sees the patient after completion of the diagnostic investigations. But at present the patients are directly consulting the specialists and super specialists neglecting the referral from family doctor or general practitioner. Failure of passing through family physician tradition has its maladies. Family physician knows better about his patient's body language, constitution, past drug history/reactions, financial status, cultural attitudes, and whims and fancies, and all these factors will play substantial role in treating a patient successfully. Specialists lack this vital information. The family is the basic unit of health care, and the patient needs individual based attention and care for which the GP is best suited.

Modern medical practice provides an opportunity to prevent illness as well as to cure the disease. Team working is an integral part of medical practice in the present era. The challenges lie in the difficulties of separating individual health care from public health care system. Service delivery is influenced by local and national policy and therefore can be subjected to rapid changes. 'Keeping up to date' through a well maintained program of continuing professional development is vital to the role of a physician.

In the early ages, medical practice was brought closer to the people by Hippocrates. He was the first physician to reject superstitions, legends, and beliefs, which credited to supernatural or divine forces that causes illness. Hippocrates was credited by the disciples of Pythagoras for allying philosophy and medicine.[1] He separated the discipline of medicine from religion, and argued that disease was not a punishment inflicted by the Gods, rather it was a product of environmental factors, diet, and living habits. Indeed, there is not a single mention of mystical illness in the entirety of the Hippocratic literature. However, Hippocrates did work with many convictions of his times.

Ancient Greek schools of medicine were split into two schools, the Knidian and Koan, on the issue of how to deal with disease. The Knidian School of medicine focused on diagnosis. Medicine, at the time of Hippocrates, knew nothing about human anatomy and physiology, because of the Greek taboo of forbidding the dissection of human corpuses. The Knidian School consequently failed to distinguish a series of symptoms caused by a single disease. The Hippocratic School and Koan School achieved greater success by applying general diagnoses and passive treatments. The focus of these schools was on patient care and prognosis, and they effectively treated diseases and contributed for the developments in clinical practice.

Hippocratic medicine and its philosophy are quite different from that of modern medicine. Now, the physician focuses on specific diagnosis and specialized treatment, both of which were espoused by the Knidian School. This shift in medical thought since Hippocrates' days has caused serious criticism. A physician is also known as a medical practitioner, medical doctor, or simply doctor, practices the ancient profession of medicine, which is concerned with maintaining or restoring human health through the study, diagnosis, and treatment of disease or injury. Medical practice properly requires both a detailed knowledge of the academic disciplines such as anatomy and physiology, underlying diseases and their treatment, the science of medicine, and also a decent competence in its applied practice, that is, the art or craft of medicine.

The role of the physician as well as the meaning of the word physician varies significantly around the world. As it is generally understood, the ethics of medicine requires that a physician should show consideration, compassion, and benevolence to their patients. The physician must not only be prepared to do what is right to him, but also make the patients, the attendants, and the externals cooperate with him. The Harrison's principles of Internal Medicine rightly state: "the patient is no mere collection of symptoms, signs, disordered functions, damaged organs, and disturbed emotions. He is human, fearful and hopeful, seeking relief and reassurance."

So a doctor may spent hours of time in examining a patient, eliciting signs and symptoms, but the patient's mind is always towards a complete relief within the least possible time, by spending a lesser amount of money. Hence, doctor's responsibility to meet the expectations of his patients is very crucial. To observe ethical norms and values, and to serve the patient to his utmost satisfaction, is the real challenge to the physicians of modern times.

Medical Ethics:

The knowledge of medical science and technology has undergone a tremendous change in the recent past. As a result of constant experimentation and innovations in the field of medical treatment the concept of ethics itself is fast changing. The new techniques invented in recent times can promote human life or relieve and prevent human suffering to a great extent. However, the progress of medical science and technology, in isolation from the overall value system of society, raises many ethical issues.

The commercialization of medical profession is increasing day by day, and it becomes a great challenge to the persons of the contemporary world. A medical professional should not consider acquisition of wealth as an end to his profession, but a means towards attaining an end. That end must be directed towards the wellbeing of the patient, and professional satisfaction of the doctor and other medical staff. A sense of contentment is essential to keep the medical professionals free from covetousness or greed for money.

Medical ethics gets its inspiration from philosophical values. In spite of rapid changes in the socio-economic fields that takes place throughout the world, certain basic ethical values have to be kept sacred for all times. It is the mission of the physician to safeguard the health of the patients. His knowledge and skills should be dedicated towards the fulfillment of this mission.

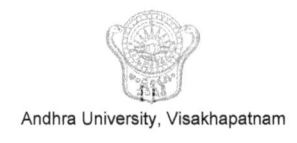

The Tasks of Medical Practice:

The ideal task of contemporary medical profession is to develop a holistic and comprehensive view of an individual patient. It is built on concepts extending from ancient Greece to the modern age. Hippocratic generalizations (460-370 BC) were clearly patient oriented. The regimen that is adopted should be for the benefit of the sick. By the late middle ages, the Jewish philosopher and physician Moses Maimonides (1135-1204), saw his task as caring for any sick person who asked his advice without any distinction between rich and poor, friend and foe, good and bad person. The second part of nineteenth century achieved many advances in understanding the epidemics of cholera, typhoid, and smallpox, which have been arose as a result of unsanitary and crowded working and living conditions. Therefore, the role of medical profession is extended to environmental controls, health education, and organizing the vaccination of children against a host of previously lethal infectious diseases, besides public health contribution. Parallel movements were occurred in Germany. Rudolf Virchow (1821-1902), the father of pathology, wrote that physicians were the natural attorneys of the poor in their struggle to solve their social problems. In the year 1974, a high level group of European Medical Practitioners met in the Dutch town of Leeuwenhorst where they produced a well accepted document that says: 'a licensed medical graduate who provides personal, primary, and continuing care to individuals, should practice his profession irrespective of age, sex and illness'. The founders of various medical theories in the history of humanity struggled to practice ethics in medicine. According to several studies carried out in Edinburgh, it is clear that it is difficult to define the quality of health care services, which is based on both critical and technical expertise. The doctor-patient relationship is an interpersonal relationship, and it is crucial to improve the quality of consultation.

Medical science and medical practitioners prevail upon to cure diseases within their limitations, relieve symptoms to the extent possible by using their talents and expertise, and comfort the patient and his family members. They are exhorted to put the interests of the patient and his family above all else. Treatment must always follow diagnosis and must use the most efficacious and least expensive means.

The medical profession is uniquely equipped to help the unfortunate sick persons for relieving pain, healing sickness to the extent possible and caring at all times. Barring a few exceptional individuals and groups, doctors in general have failed in their duties to the clints.[6]

The present state of medical practice in India fills the observer with a sense of dismay. In most of the physicians, the urge to help or serve the patients has been replaced by a compelling drive to gain immense wealth in the shortest possible period. A senior physician rightly said: "Medicine is no more called a vocation. It has become just another form of commerce or business."[7]

Being a researcher in the area of HIV/AIDS, I was so curious about the mysterious nature of AIDS from the day it has come to light and I am continuing my unending journey to explore it since 1984. When I was doing research in Andhra Medical College and King George Hospital, Visakhapatnam, on Hepatitis B, I was fascinated to study on AIDS, as it has the same mode of spread as that of Hepatitis B, i.e. through sex with an infected person, through contaminated needle, through infected blood and to a child from its HIV positive mother.

Subsequently, in the year 1987, I got an opportunity to attend a conference namely "caring for AIDS" in London at the invitation of the Royal Society of Health (UK). After a strong endeavor, I got an opportunity to see for the first time the AIDS patients in my life at Manchester Infirmary. From that time onwards I have been encountering several social, cultural, and ethical issues involved in AIDS, and interacting personally with thousands of AIDS patients, both AIDS infected and AIDS affected.

As a physician, I am deeply involved in the mission of treating AIDS patients; and also as an activist I am struggling to protect the Human Rights of PLWAS (People Living With AIDS); and as a social worker and responsible citizen I am working towards creating awareness on AIDS in the community and to prevent its spread; and as a researcher I am working to discover the best therapeutic modules, evolving newer modalities and strategies to make human society free of AIDS. The subject of AIDS is so close to my heart, and most of my time is being dedicated for the cause of HIV/AIDS. I feel that no disease in the history of medicine has created so much horror, panic, discrimination, stigma, violation of human rights, psychological trauma; and social, political, economic, religious, and ethical problems as HIV/AIDS caused. The HIV infection has already taken deep roots in India, and if it is left unchecked, the alarming spread will be a great threat to a developing country like ours.[8]

Under this background the present work, "Ethical Challenges Involved in the Treatment and Control of HIV/AIDS – An Analytical Study in Medical Ethics" is an original work based on my personal clinical experience, and scientific study of several facets of AIDS. As a practicing physician, if my knowledge goes correct, the present work is a unique thesis in the area of medical ethics.

The thesis consists of eight chapters including introduction and conclusion. To avoid repetition of ideas, I would like to mention briefly the subject matter discussed in each of these chapters.

The first and introductory chapter includes medical profession and its relation to ethics from ancient Greece to modern times, the tasks of medical profession, and the subject matter discussed in other chapters of the thesis.

The Second chapter deals with ethical theories and principles, especially the ethical theories and principles that are applicable or relevant to medical practice. It refers to ethical theories such as consequential, deontological and virtue ethics. It includes the nature of professional ethics, doctor–patient relationship, principles of beneficence and nonmaleficence, rights of patients and duties of the doctors, human dignity and autonomy, truth telling and confidentiality, informed consent, the nature of professional ethics, the purpose of health care system, the role of surrogates in decision making, corporate hospitals, the role of hospital ethics committees, and so on.

In the third chapter, I have discussed about the history of HIV/AIDS and the controversies surrounding the discovery of HIV, the origin of HIV, the methods of AIDS screening, the misconceptions surrounding AIDS tests, problems in response to false positive and false negative HIV test results, ethical problems involved in mass screening, HIV testing before marriage and the moral issues and dilemmas involved in them. Also HIV testing during pregnancy, the social predicaments to the children born to HIV positive parents, the difficulties to beget children by HIV positive couple and its consequences are discussed.

The fourth chapter deals with AIDS and legal disputes, the complex problems faced by the AIDS patients in their work places, homosexuality, and law, landmark judgment of Delhi High Court on homosexuality and some reactions of religious leaders, spread of HIV, gay sex and human rights, sexual behaviour of truck drivers, the moral issues arising in employing HIV positive persons, moral responsibilities of the HIV infected and their behaviour, condom use and ethical issues, Pope's comments on condom use, Microbicides, Catholic Bishop's acceptance to the use of condoms, unethical vengeance, chastity and religious beliefs, ethical issues related to HIV prevention, and difference of opinion involved in the legal problems.

The fifth chapter explains the practical problems of AIDS care and ethical challenges, the troubles faced by physicians and other health care providers in treating AIDS patients, the social stigma attached to AIDS treating centers, and the societal perception towards HIV physicians and AIDS patients, advertisements for AIDS treatment, HIV positive health care persons, HIV risk for health care professionals, WHO's study and use of unsafe injections, guidelines on ethical aspects of HIV infection, duties and rights of doctors infected with HIV, HIV testing regulations, and ethical problems involved in giving information to the patient's spouse.

The sixth chapter discusses about the scourge of 21st century AIDS stigma and discrimination of AIDS patients, the moral confrontations of the patients in every day life, ethics of care, judiciary and their colleagues living with HIV/AIDS, gender and stigma, AIDS ambassadors to fight on stigma, schools for HIV infected children, social issues, women and HIV/AIDS, approach to an HIV positive patient, human rights and HIV/AIDS, and the right to private and family life.

In the seventh chapter, I have honestly presented, my research findings in AIDS and ethics, AIDS drugs and vaccine trials conducted in India and ethical benchmarks, principle of essentiality, principles of non-exploitation, informed consent, principles of privacy and confidentiality, principles of precaution and risk minimization, principles of professional competence, principles of accountability and transparency, principles of maximization of the public interest and distributive justice, principles of institutional arrangements, public domain, totality of responsibility and principles of compliance, the HIV/AIDS and health insurance, different types of insurance policies, death futures, insurance coverage problems to HIV patients, improving the quality of death, the millennium development goals, budding health/life insurance for people living with HIV/AIDS in India, internationally protected human rights such as the right to life and survival, the right to health care, the right to liberty and security of the person, the right to freedom from torture or ill-treatment, the right to marry and found a family and other human rights issues in the wake of UNO declaration.

In the eighth and conclusion chapter, I have discussed about the changing trends of HIV/AIDS treatment and its modern management, the fall of glory of medical profession and suggestions to regain the past magnificence, code of ethics for medical practice, ethical issues related to AIDS orphans, negligence of media about right reporting of HIV/AIDS stories, press council of India guidelines for media coverage, unethical reports about AIDS, psychological support, home based care and moral issues, Tanzanian model, prostitution and AIDS, ethics of family system, legalization of homosexuality and its impact on HIV/AIDS, lesbians and ethical viewpoints, AIDS in jails and armed forces, solutions suggested to prevent AIDS, and a critical analysis of medical practice and decline of ethical values, how to regain the past glory, and various dilemmas in the era of AIDS have been portrayed.

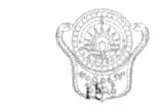

Andhra University, Visakhapatnam

References:

1. Douglas Wilson and Mark Cotton (eds), *"Handbook of HIV Medicine"* (New York, Oxford University press, 2010), pp.3–9.

2. Madhu Gurung, *"NACO News"* Vol.5, Issue I, (New Delhi, New Concept International Systems Pvt. Ltd., with support from UNDP, 2010), pp. 4-5

3. www.wisdomquotes.com, *"humanism quotes"*. Google search

4. Albert R. Jonsen, Mark Siegler and William J. Winslade, *"Clinical Ethics: A Practical Approach to Ethical Decisions in Clinical Medicine"*, (New York: McGraw Hill, 1998), p. 145

5. James H. Rutherford, *"Moral and Political Philosophy"*, (Columbus, Top 20 Publishing Co., 2004), pp. 139-140

6. S.K. Pandya, *"National Seminar on Bioethics"*, (Bombay, Joshi Bedekar College, Thane, 2007) pp.1-2.

7. Sunil K. Pandya *"Mans Sana Monographs"*, (Mumbai, Jaslok Hospital and research centre, 2006), pp. 50-61.

8. Kutikuppala Surya Rao, Editor's choice: "Epidemic Kaposi's sarcoma in AIDS- A General Overview" – *"Journal of Applied Medicine"*, (London, Northwood Publications), p. 137,

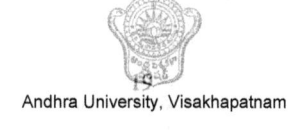

@@@@@

Chapter Two

Ethical Theories and Principles Relevant to Medical Profession

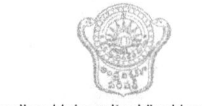

Andhra University, Visakhapatnam

CHAPTER – II

ETHICAL THEORIES AND PRINCIPLES RELEVANT TO MEDICAL PROFESSION

Ethics has been described as the science of morals or rules of conduct concerning human life. Ethics is a branch of philosophy, which is also called as moral philosophy. Ethics is a normative science that studies about the good and bad, right and wrong actions of individuals and institutions. In ethics the terms "right" and "wrong" apply only to the acts of a person, whereas "good" and "bad" refers to the results of acts, the motives from which the act was done, the intention of the person carrying out the deed, and the person who is the agent of a particular act.

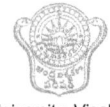

Since ethics is rooted in reason, it does not depend on religious beliefs as a source of its conclusions. Philosophers like Aristotle and Kant regarded ethics as a rational enterprise, which means that it is based on reason, rather than religious beliefs or personal feelings and impulses. Ethics is rational also means that human beings are autonomous moral agents, who can decide for themselves what they ought to do, or ought not to do, and justify their actions on the basis of reasons, and hold responsibility to the consequences of their actions.[1]

When we apply the principles of ethics to a particular profession, it becomes necessary to discuss not only about the basic standards of those ethical theories, but also about the nature of the profession, and the conditions under which that profession operates. Now, let us discuss about some ethical theories and principles that are relevant to medical profession.

Ethical theories propose some principle or principles to differentiate right actions from wrong actions. These theories can be broadly divided into three classes — consequential, deontological and virtue ethics.

Consequential Theories:

Many philosophers have argued that the moral rightness of an action is determined by its results. If its consequences are good, then the act is right, and if they are bad, the act is wrong. Moral theories which adopt this approach are called consequential theories.

The consequential theories judge the rightness or the wrongness of an action on the basis of the consequences brought about by that action. The consequences are evaluated on the basis of some intrinsic good that they serve, or that is something good in and of itself without any further consequences. For example, utilitarianism is a form of consequential theory, which holds that an action is good if it yields the greatest amount of pleasure to the greatest number of people and least amount of pain. The principle of "utility" is the basic moral principle of utilitarianism. Accordingly, right actions are those that produce the best consequences, or intended to produce grater amount of good over evil.[2]

Utilitarian principle has certain difficulties in the field of medical ethics for the following reasons:

1) It overlooks the good of the individual and concentrates more on the greatest good of greatest number of people.
2) Since this theory is forward looking in its evaluation, the consequences of an action are not clear enough to be accurately measured and evaluated in a systematic way.
3) The consequences of certain actions are unforeseeable, and hence, they are not clear to judge in a rightful way.

Deontological Theories:

Deontology, as an ethical theory, determines the rightness or wrongness of an action on the basis of certain characteristics of the action such as – duty, justice, intention, respect for individual dignity and autonomy etc. Unlike consequential theory, deontological theory considers certain acts as good or evil in and of themselves irrespective of their consequences. For example, lying is wrong for a deontologist like Kant, even if a lie would produce greatest good for the individual or society. In judging the rightness of an act, the deontologist uses certain ethical principles or rules such as: "Do unto others as you would have them do unto you" or "Act in such a way that you always treat humanity as an end, but never as a means." For the deontologist, an action is morally right if it has been done with good intention or with a sense of duty or with a respect to the dignity of persons. For Kant, the moral worth of an action depends on its intention, but not on its consequences.[3]

One of the strengths of deontological theory is its emphasis on the moral significance of the individual. But it gives less importance to the community. Our experiences with friendship, marriage and community living indicate that these realities are central in the moral development and moral life of the individual. Indeed, society is the means by which the individual develops his reason and trained to social roles. Any position that does not give a proper place to the fundamental moral relationship between the individual and society seems to be inadequate.

Virtue Ethics:

The moral philosophy that concentrates on the concept of virtue is called virtue ethics .Virtue ethics refers to the traits of character that makes human behaviour praiseworthy or blameworthy. It involves not only the virtues, but also the integration of virtues with practical wisdom or right reason. Virtues are good traits, and a virtuous person is a morally good person. For virtue ethics, the moral life is about developing good character. For example, if we consider honesty or truthfulness as ideals, then we ought to try to become honest and truthful persons. The opposite of virtue is vice. Here the moral praise or blame focuses on the virtues or vices of the people concerned, but not on the results of their actions.

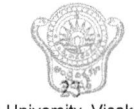

Instead of enquiring about whether a particular action is right or wrong, virtue ethics asks what virtues or qualities a person should possess if he lives the good life? Virtues are those qualities that can enable someone to live well and fulfill himself as a human being. Though there are various virtues, the ancient Greeks identified four virtues as cardinal virtues – temperance, justice, courage and prudence (practical wisdom).

For Aristotle, virtue is in harmony with one's nature, whereas vice is in disharmony with it. Man's essential nature is the actualization of his potentialities. Virtue is an excellence of some sort. Moral virtue is a state of character and it is within man's power to cultivate. Moral virtues are not learned by teaching, but are developed by practice.[4] For instance, by practicing courage, we become more courageous; by practicing honesty we become more honest. Moral virtue implies choice, and choice implies rational deliberation, which is a unique quality of human beings. Man acts voluntarily in the sense that he has the rational power or reflective thinking to do or not to do certain things.[5]

Applied Ethics:

Ethical theories by themselves are not adequate to solve moral problems at the practical level. Ethics is not merely a theoretical study, but also an application of moral principles and standards to particular kinds of cases of practical life, to evaluate and justify human and institutional actions, as right or wrong, moral or immoral.

Ethical inquiry is of two kinds, theoretical and practical. The question "what is morality?" is different from the question "what should I do?" The first question refers to the meaning of morality, and the second question refers to the practical aspect of morality.

Thus, applied ethics is distinguished from theoretical ethics by its special focus on issues of practical concern and controversies, rather than questions of ethical theory. In fact, theoretical ethics and applied ethics are not completely separate from one another, but lie on a continuum from the abstract to the concrete.

Applied ethics includes a wide range of issues covering medical ethics, business ethics, environmental ethics, and so on. But, the present work is confined to medical ethics, especially to the ethical problems arise from the treatment of HIV/AIDS and other attendant issues attached to it.

The Nature of Professional Ethics:

Professional ethics is a special type of applied ethics. There are different views about the nature of professional ethics.

1. First, a set of rules might be called professional ethics because the members of a particular profession articulate it.
2. Secondly, it is concerned with the ethical conduct of the profession.

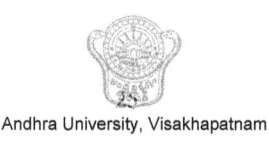

The first type of professional ethics is found in the codes of ethics promulgated by the professional group. These rules are supposed to govern the conduct of members of a given profession. Many thinkers thought that an uncritical acceptance of every provision of the professional codes is not wise.

In professional ethics the role definition of a person is crucial. It determines what duties are specific to the members of the profession, and which rights will be granted by the society. Every profession has specific obligations that depend on what is approved as the purpose of the profession within the culture. For example, a profession like law is set up and approved for the promotion of justice according to the constitution and laws of a specific society. Thus, the lawyer has a duty to represent the interests of his clients in order to ensure a fair trail even though that might result in some perpetrators of crimes going free.

The Physician-Patient Relationship:

What should be the relationship between Physician and patient? The Physician-patient relationship may be explained from three different viewpoints – paternalism, individualism and reciprocal or collegial. [6]

Paternalism:

Paternalism is a position which says that health care professionals should take a parental role towards patients. According to this position, the health care professionals possess a superior knowledge of medicine and specialized training, and thus they alone could decide what is best for the patients. This attitude refers to the traditional idea of "the doctor always knows the best". A number of arguments are put forth to support this viewpoint:

1. The nonprofessional people lack the professional knowledge and expertise of medicine, and therefore, they cannot decide what is best for the patients.
2. The Professionals, because of their knowledge and long experience, know the characteristics of diseases and the necessary treatment, and therefore, the patients should trust the knowledge of professionals and leave all matters relating to the treatment to them.
3. All decisions about patient's care and treatment should be in the hands of doctors, and the patient should not interfere with the treatment suggested by doctors.

Individualism:

Individualism is the position that supports patient's rights over their own bodies and lives. There are a number of arguments supporting this position.

1. Doctors, like any other human being, are capable of committing errors in judgment, diagnosis, prognosis, and treatment. At times, they are guilty of negligence and malpractice or maltreatment.
2. The patients or their family members are the best judges to decide what kind of treatment is to be given under the existing medical condition and circumstances.
3. The patient or his lawful surrogate should decide whether a particular treatment is beneficial to the patient or not in the given situation.

4. Paternalism has often led to total dependence of the patient on the doctor, ignoring that the patient is a person who can take rational decisions about what is good for him, whether he should or should not take the treatment suggested by the doctor.

The Reciprocal or Collegial:

This position involves a team approach to treatment that includes patients and their family members on one hand and health care providers on the other, who work together and do what is best to the patient. This position is supported on the following arguments.

1. It is important to recognize the rights of individual patients to make free choices concerning their treatment since it is their bodies and lives which are at stake. Even if the rights of the patients are not absolute they should be given high priority.

2. Patients have the right to information about their diagnosis, treatment, respectful care, and prognosis; need to give informed consent to any procedure with full knowledge about human experimentation and the right to refuse it.

3. Neither the patients nor health care providers alone know best, but decisions involving treatment are to be reciprocal (involving give and take) and collegial (involving group approach in decision making). Thus all decisions being made jointly by patients and their doctors.

4. Patients are entitled to more than one professional opinion that is to be appraised of all the expertise that can be brought to bear on their cases so that they can make important decisions.

5. All decisions about treatment should be arrived at through the exchange of ideas and a full discussion of alternative methods of treatment.

The Principles of Beneficence and Nonmaleficence:

The principle of beneficence asserts "doing good" to every individual, and the principle of nonmaleficence requires "avoiding evil" to all persons. Thus, these two principles directly refer to the Hippocrates oath, which is obligatory to every medical practitioner. At the time of taking the oath, the doctor declares: "I will use treatment to help the sick according to my ability and judgment, but never with a view to injury and wrong doing." The Hippocrates oath prescribes certain codes of behaviour to medical practitioners and it forbids doing harm to any patient. In the context of medical treatment "doing good" means taking certain actions which benefits the patient.

The Dignity of the Individual:

Human beings have an intrinsic worth or dignity which, makes them valuable above all else. Since human beings are rational beings, they must be treated with respect. Individuals should not be used as mere things or objects and manipulated to achieve one's own ends. We must always recognize and respect humanity in others. Therefore, humans should not be used as a means to an end. The principle of the golden rule says: "treat others only in ways that we would be willing to be treated ourselves."

According to Kant, human dignity requires treating individual persons with respect in whom that dignity resides. We may use the services of others and benefit from their actions, but we must not violate their dignity as persons. For example, slavery is morally wrong because it treats people as commodities, and it fails to give proper respect to the personhood of the slave. In the context of medical profession, human dignity implies that each person should determine his own destiny and the health care professionals should not violate the patient's right to self-determination. The demands of human dignity are crucial in medical ethics, especially in the consideration of truth telling and informed consent.

The concept of human dignity is not a static concept. The history of humanity shows how this concept has been changed from time to time. For example, at different times of history, the human society recognized the evils of slavery, sexism, racism, ageism, child labour and the like as affronts to human dignity. To practice such social evils is a great insult to human dignity. Sometimes the societies are tempted to down grade the dignity of the sick, elderly, poor, and powerless due to selfishness or shortsightedness.

The Principle of Autonomy:

The dignity of the person commands to respect individual persons. In other words, respect for the dignity of the individual involves not only leaving people alone to make their own choices, but also recognizing that no individual has the right to touch another without his or her consent. It implies that one human being does not have authority or power over another human being. Hence, no person should coerce others, or limit their activities, or impose their will on others. Even the government or social institutions must respect the freedom and privacy of individuals, and they may interfere only when it is necessary to protect the dignity of others, or when there are overriding social concerns.

Since the respect for freedom and privacy ultimately rooted in the dignity of a person, the principle of autonomy calls for respecting even those persons who are unconscious or in a coma. Even the non-autonomous person is to be respected for the reason that persons are intrinsically valuable in and of themselves, not because of any other consideration such as they are useful to society or highly intelligent or possess exemplary qualities. Hence, no individual person should be used or treated as a thing.

The respect for persons, in general, and their freedom, in particular, has consequences for all professions. For example, neither doctors nor nurses have a right to interfere with individuals, or force their opinions on them, or even act on a person's behalf without permission. The principle of autonomy, more accurately, the principle of patient's autonomy is the core of medical ethics.

In the medical profession, the principle of autonomy expresses the view: "you shall not treat a patient without the informed consent of the patient or his lawful surrogate, except in certain emergencies." This principle clarifies the meaning of respect for the person and his freedom in the context of health care. It not only seeks to prevent medical tyranny, but also aims autonomous decision-making by the patient.

Informed Consent:

The term "informed consent" refers to a formal procedure whereby the patients or their lawful surrogates (when patients are incapacitated) give consent in writing to some sort of medical treatment, procedure or surgery, which may have some side effects, and affect patients' future lives or even involve the risk of death.

Informed consent means telling truth to the patient about his illness, and involving him making decisions in an autonomous way concerning the treatment. This approach became necessary in recent times because many technological tests involve painful and risky procedures and surgeries required in the treatment of patients. The patients should be informed fully, what is to be done, why it is to be done, when it is to be done, and what amount of pain, discomfort or risk is involved in the treatment. Except in emergency situations, wherein saving a life requires immediate action, patients or their lawful surrogates must authorize any procedure of serious nature, such as surgeries, certain kinds of laboratory tests and therapies.[7]

The concept of informed consent is a crucial concept in medical practice. It is relatively a new concept in medical ethics. Many traditional health care professionals believe that certain things need not be informed to the patient, but to be concealed from him. They did not seek consent of patients, but try to control them. For example, Hippocrates, after whom "Hippocratic Oath" is named, thought that most things should be concealed from patients while caring for them. Nothing should be told to the patients about their present or future condition. The concept of informed consent raises the following questions:

1. Is informed consent an aid or impediment to good medical care?
2. Is physician's intervention in the lives of his patients require justification?
3. What grounds adequately justify paternalistic intervention in the life of another?

In recent times, many democratic governments all over the world brought some changes in law, and as a result of those changes, informed consent becomes a necessary component of health care. Since the patient is a full participant in the healing process, he or she should be informed fully about the risks involved in treatment or surgery. Hence, to disregard informed consent is to risk lawsuits, and in such cases the health care professionals should take responsibility of their invasive procedures. Informed consent involves the following conditions:

1. The patient or an appropriate lawful surrogate, who has a capacity for decision making, who is capable of understanding the consequences of the consent, and who is free from coercion and undue influence comes under informed consent.
2. The health care professionals, within the demands of their particular role, must provide the necessary information to the patient and made sure that it is understood.

In general, if any one of these condition is not present, then, there is no informed consent of the patient and so no authorization of treatment. The health care professional does not have a right to treat the patient who is incompetent to give his or her consent because he or she is unconscious or severely injured or mentally retarded. Since the effect of the treatment involves the patient's health, life, lifestyle, values, and religious beliefs, the physician should take decision of the patient or the lawful surrogate, to accept or reject a particular treatment.

Sometimes the patient may prefer to suffer the pain from the disease rather than the pain from the treatment. The patient may prefer to die rather than put the family through a long agony that leaves them in emotionally drained and financially overburdened state. Hence, the health care professionals must resist the temptation to impose their values, that is, the value of health and life on patients.

Exceptions to Informed Consent:

The obligation to obtain informed consent before proceeding to treat a patient is exempted for emergency cases. To justify emergency treatment without informed consent should include the following three conditions.

1. The patient must be incapable of giving consent, and no lawful surrogate is available at that time to give consent.
2. There is a danger of life or danger of a serious impairment of health.
3. Immediate treatment is necessary to avert those dangers.

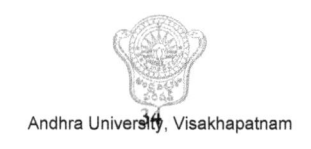

Therapeutic Privilege and Concealment of Information:

Physicians have long claimed, and the law has often recognized, an exception called the therapeutic privilege.[8] Therapeutic privilege is the privilege of withholding information from the patient when the physician believes the disclosure will have an adverse effect on the patient's condition or health. Those who justify this privilege must limit it by placing the following three conditions on its use.

1. The actual use of the privilege must not be based on generalities, but on the actual circumstances of the patient, or on a **case-by-case basis**.
2. The mere fact that the patient will be disturbed by bad news is not a sufficient justification for the use of the privilege. The physician must have an intimate knowledge about the patient, and the must be convinced that the full disclosure will have a significant adverse effect on him.
3. The physician may not be justified in concealing all the information. He should use reasonable discretion in the manner and extent of the disclosure.

The serious problem involved in the therapeutic privilege is its denial of patient's autonomy.

Patient's Right to Refuse Treatment:

The doctrine of individual autonomy clearly implies that the patient or the surrogate has a right to refuse treatment. This right does not depend on whether or not the refusal of treatment can make good sense to someone else, but only on the competence of the patient. Even in a psychiatric facility, the result to refuse treatment remains unless ordered by a court. The right to refuse does not imply that the patient is ethical in refusing treatment, but health care provider is not ethical in forcing treatment on the patient or treating the patient without informed consent. The American Hospital Association's Bill of patient's Rights summarizes this right as follows:

"The patient has the right to refuse treatment to the extent permitted by law and to be informed of the medical consequences of his actions".

Principles of Truthfulness and Confidentiality:

The issue of truth telling involves, to what extent the patients or their lawful surrogate should be told the truth about their illness or dying.

In a discussion about patients' and professionals' rights and obligations, there are two views of truth telling in medicine the paternalistic view and the patients' right to know.

The Paternalistic View of Truth Telling:

There are several arguments put forth to support the paternalistic viewpoint.

1. Since the patients are not medically trained, they do not need to know more than the fact that the professionals will do their best to them.

2. It is good for the patients, if they are not told the truth, especially if it is bad news, because the knowledge about such condition

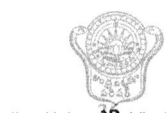

might cause anxiety in them and consequently they cannot fight for their survival.

3. If the prognosis is that they are going to die, it would serve no purpose to tell them bad news, so that they live as happily as they can for the remaining period before death.

4. It may be appropriate to tell the bad news to his family members, but not the patients, for patients should be protected from bad news.

5. The health care providers as well as the family members of the patients should not discuss the seriousness of patients' illness, injuries or dying with the patient. Everyone should try to cheer them up and avoid bad news wherever it is possible.

The Patients' Right to Know:

There are a number of arguments in support of patients' right to know about the diagnosis and the proposed treatment to cure illness.

1. Since it is patients', bodies and lives that are involved, not those of health care providers, patients have a right to know everything concerning the disease and the proposed treatment, and it is the duty of the physicians to tell all information to the patients.

2. If the patients know everything what is going on concerning the treatment, it is much easier to the physicians to treat them and get the expected results of their treatment.

3. Patients are often angry or disappointed if they do not know about the side effects or painful treatment or disturbing aspects of treatment.

The Moderate Position:

This view lies between paternalism and frankness of the physicians in sharing appropriate information with the patients when they want to know it. It involves the following aspects.

1. The physician should listen to the patients carefully and try to understand what the patients really want to know from them.
2. The physician must try to answer all the questions and doubts raised by the patients truthfully, yet not brutally.
3. The physician should reveal the bad news to the patient not at once, but in gradual doses or installment wise to avoid the shock of bad news.
4. The physician should tell the truth gently, clearly, and humanely, never hopelessly or cruelly.
5. The physician should try to explain to the patient everything in simple terms, but not using technical and medical language that the patient unable to understand.

In medical profession, as in the case of other professions, the health care providers should fallow the principles of truthfulness and confidentiality. Telling truth is a difficult problem, and sometimes it may lead to disaster consequences. Telling truth does not mean as telling the whole truth. Some truth should be kept confidential. But it is difficult to decide what truth may be concealed and what truth must be revealed.

The health care provider must provide the basic truths to the patient or his surrogate in order to get informed consent. The patient had a right to the information and thus the physician had an obligation to communicate it to him. The doctrine of informed consent, however, does not cover all the problems of truthfulness. For example, should a physician write on a death certificate that the patient died of AIDS? In certain situations the truth ought to be kept confidential or concealed from people other than the patient. For example, should the physician conceal from a wife the fact that her husband has herpes? When can a physician reveal sensitive information to a nurse or another physician?

The ethics of truthfulness may be summed up in two commands:
1. When you are communicating, do not lie.
2. You must communicate truth with those who have a right to the truth.

Neither of the two commands says that you must tell everyone everything you know or everything that they want to know. The first command leaves you free not to communicate, by remaining silent or evading the question or tells a falsehood, which is not the same thing as a lie. The second command raises the question of who has a right to communication of truth.

Lying:

A lie may be defined as a communicative expression of a falsehood to the other person, who has a reasonable expectation of the truth. One need not communicate truth, if someone enquires about very private matters such as one's finances, sex life, or health problems etc., To conceal truth is not a lie, though it may be unethical for other reasons. By keeping silent or by evading the question people used to avoid telling truth. It would be quite different to tell falsehood to a person who enquires about the way to a hospital or a bus station. There is no reason for keeping such things concealed, when the other person has reasonable expectation of the truth.

However, the patient who goes to a physician for a diagnosis has a reasonable expectation of truth from the physician. Similarly, a physician who is preparing a health history of a patient would have a reasonable expectation of truthful answers to all questions bearing on diagnosis.

The Right of a Person to the Truth:

The right to truth involves two kinds of truthful information.

1. The patient has a right to the information necessary for informed consent because he has to take decisions about treatment.
2. In some cases other than treatment, the patient may have a right to truthful information because he may have a right to the truth by purchase. For example, if a person goes to a health provider, not to treatment but to know the condition of blood pressure, he has a right to the truth because he paid for it.

Therefore, it is ethically wrong to tell falsehood in those situations where there is a reasonable expectation of the truth. The expectation of truth varies with the persons to be communicated and the nature of the material to be communicated. We have an obligation to communicate truth only when the person has a right to the information as a result of contract or relationship. Hence, it is wrong to tell falsehood where the person has right to the truth, and also in the situations where persons have reasonable expectations of the truth.

Confidentiality:

The same sets of obligations that are discussed in the context of truthfulness are also applicable with regard to confidentiality when the health care providers deal with families and other third parties about the condition of the patients.

Confidentiality is concerned with keeping things secret. A secret is knowledge about a person, and the health care provider has an obligation to conceal it. The obligation to keep secrets arises from the fact that if a particular knowledge is revealed it will harm the person concerned. The professional secret if revealed, not only harm the client of that professional but also damage the image of that profession.

Professional secrets, in general, need not be revealed even in courts. A physician need not disclose information learned in confidence from his patient unless the patient gives his permission. Thus, the professional secret is the most serious of all secrets, because its violation can cause great harm. The healthcare professionals are expected to maintain confidentiality for the following reasons.

Sometimes the harm that comes from concealing a natural secret outweighs the harm that is to be avoided. In such cases proportionality justifies revelation, and also makes it a duty. For example, if you know a person with AIDS tries to donate blood to some blood bank, then you have a proportionate reason to tell the in charge of the blood bank about his condition in order to prevent harm to the recipients of his blood. Where there is no foreseeable harm, you could not be justified in revealing the natural secret.

A secret that is promised to conceal should not be revealed unless that promised secret has some harmful effects to other persons. Since social life depends on people keeping promises, revealing a promised secret makes breaking of the promises, and in such cases people distrust one another. As in the case of natural secret, there may be proportionate reason for revealing the secret. The good to be attained must outweigh the evil that results from the broken promise.

For example, a man infected with the AIDS virus insists that his condition be kept confidential, even from his wife. The doctor's moral duty does not require that the patient's request for confidentiality be hanoured. Here the duty of the doctor to his patient is only a prima-facie duty that can be overridden by stronger moral duties such as the duty not to harm others.

People, in general, do not want to tell their secrets to someone who cannot be trusted to keep a secret. Indeed, the patient-physician relationship implies a promise of secrecy. People feel that the condition of their body is private and to be shared with only those they choose to help them, but not with others. For this reason, the health care providers must observe secrecy in order to keep their services acceptable to the people who need them.

Society has long recognized the importance of professional secrecy for the following reasons.

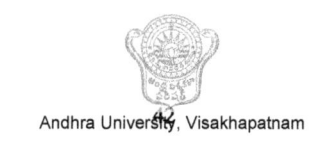

1. The patient has the right to privacy concerning case discussion, consultation, examination and treatment, and therefore, all health care professionals are expected to maintain confidentiality.
2. The patient has the right to expect that all communications and records pertaining to his or her care are confidential.

Although the medical records are made primarily for the good of the patient, they also provide a valuable source of information for medical research. The records should not be used without the informed consent of the patient. A medical researcher should be kept two things in mind to protect confidentiality.

1. When publishing his research papers or research results, he should publish only summary data of records with no identification of persons.
2. The number of people who see the medical record should be kept to minimum.

The introduction of third-party payers or health insurance into the health care system has weakened confidentiality. Whenever the physician or hospital applies for reimbursement of medical expenses through our insurance policy, we will give permission for the non-professional employees to supply information about our diagnosis and treatment to the insurance company. At the insurance company this information is handled by clerks and fed into a computer.

The information about our health that came into the hands of life insurers or employers may have harmful consequences. For example, if the treatment relates for a mental condition of a person, his or her chances for promotion to a higher position might be affected. Thus, the computerization of health care information causes a potential harm to patients.

Moral and Legal Rights:

Social ethics can be known through the constitution of a nation, which speaks of the rights of individuals such as the right to life, liberty, and the pursuit of happiness. Sometimes, the term "right" is no more than a means of expressing a set of ideals or goals for human development. For example, the United Nations Universal Declaration of Human Rights (1948) is best understood as an expression of hopes, rather than realities.

In the discussion of ethics, the term "right" is used as a moral or legal claim that an individual may assert against someone else. Thus, there are two types of rights, moral rights, in which the claim is based on moral principles, and legal rights, in which the claim is based on law. Any such claim imposes an obligation on another person. A legal right may be asserted when the appropriate legislation has been made law, or when a judicial decision confirms an interpretation of law. Thus, legal rights are derived from the legal system of the state.

In addition to legal rights, there are certain moral or human rights, which are naturally conferred to all individuals by virtue of being that they are human beings. Human rights do not depend on the legal system of a state the way legal rights depend. The law may protect human rights, but the law is not the source of human rights.

There are two types of human rights negative and positive. The right to life, liberty and pursuit of happiness are negative rights, where others should not interfere with these rights in certain ways. For example, it is morally wrong to take away the right to life of a person, even if doing so maximizes the social good. But, if someone violates the right to life of another, then he looses his right to life, and he would be punished according to the legal system of the state.

In contrast to negative rights, the positive human rights refer to the vital interests of the human beings in getting certain benefits from others. For example, positive rights include the right to health, education, employment, and so on.

In the context of medical profession, the patients' rights impose restrictions on the health care professionals not to interfere with their rights, even to do good to them. Thus, the health care professionals should respect the freedom of the patients and get informed consent of the patients before they start the proposed treatment or surgery.

The Role of Surrogates in Decision Making:

Surrogates are people who are authorized by law or custom to make decisions when the patient is incompetent to make his own decision. Surrogates have an important role in health care ethics.

Ordinarily, parents are considered as surrogates for their minor children, spouses for one another, adult children for parents or grandparents, parents or grandparents for grandchildren, brothers and sisters, and uncles and aunts, the patient's family friends or their relatives are believed to know the desires and values of the patient, and are trusted to act in the best interest of the patient.

In some cases, a difficult situation may arise to the health care providers due to difference of opinion among two or more potential surrogates. For example, the surrogate may want the patient to die in order to make his life easier, but the patient could have a reasonable life if treated well. In such cases, the health care professional may know what the patient desired ignoring the decision of the surrogate, because the surrogates should not always have the last word. The health care professional in the cases of life and death matters, must proceed with caution, and if necessary, seek court intervention when he believes that the best interests of the patient are being neglected.

Who should inform the Patient or the Surrogates?

Most writers on medical ethics maintain that it is the primary responsibility of the physician to inform the patient or surrogate. The hospitals and other health care institutions have at least supervisory responsibility to make sure that their employees have informed the patient. When the patient asks what is going on, what drug is being administered, what are its side effects, these questions should be answered within the limits of the expertise of the particular health care provider.

The report of the American Hospital's committee on Biomedical Ethics notes the following obligations of the hospital with regard to informed consent:

1. To ensure that informed consent has been obtained for diagnostic and therapeutic procedures performed in the hospital.
2. To develop educational programs that teaches effective ways of getting ethically and legally acceptable informed consent.
3. To make certain that patients are aware of their right to consent or reject proposed procedures and treatments.

The Health Care Profession:

Membership in a profession brings with it obligations specific to that profession or the roles they play in that profession. The roles assigned to health care workers change from society to society and from time to time, because they are influenced by the value system of a given society as well as by the goals and aspirations of the profession. For example, the Hippocratic tradition paternalistically saw the physician in charge of everything. In recent times, under the influence of the Western liberal political tradition, changes occurred in health care system resulting in the recognition of patient's rights and societal obligations. For health care professionals, the primary ethical consideration is protecting the dignity of the individual human person.

The Purpose of Health Care System:

The primary purpose of health care system is the prevention of disease and the maintenance of health of the individuals. In the medical profession there are some problems that have ethical implications. Since the value of life and the prolongation of life involve contradictory ethical positions, there are three conflicting views about the purpose of health care system.

1. If the purpose of health care is the prevention of death, then the physicians are professionally correct when they keep people alive even though in a vegetative state.
2. If the purpose is the relief of suffering by either cure or care, the physician who uses certain "innovative measures" with a person in a permanent vegetative state is cruel and unprofessional.
3. If the purpose is to optimize the patient's chances for a happy and productive life, then the treatment that dooms the patient to an unproductive life is perhaps unethical.

Corporate Hospitals:

In recent times, the physician-patient relationship as a personal and professional relationship is changed due to the advent of corporate hospitals, where the physician works as a businessman and the hospital as a business firm with serious consequences for both health care system and health care ethics.

When the patient and the physician have developed a clearly personal relationship, then, each knows the values of the others, and they share mutual trust. Hence, personal relationship between the patient and the physician is thought to be an ideal relationship.

Health care providers of corporate hospitals are increasingly rush for customers, employing marketing strategies, and attempting to increase their profits. This type of trend changed the public image of doctors and hospitals. The new economic orientation, as well as the increase in the number of physicians created a new tendency among the physicians to do more for each patient in order to earn more income. Thus, the new emerging trend turned the physician into a tradesman.

The Role of Hospital Ethics Committees:

Hospital Ethics Committee (HEC) is formed in the health care centers with multidisciplinary groups of health care professionals and community representatives to educate about medical ethics, to help in policy development, and to act as consultants in difficult cases. Although the legal status of these committees is not very clear, the courts in general will respect the recommendations of these committees. The HEC acts as a mediator in resolving conflicts and dilemmas about patient care.

Although the role of the HEC is admirable, some cautions seem to be necessary in its functioning.

1. Since the goals of the committee are not always clear, some committees that are dominated by health care professionals, extend their support to health care professionals or reducing their legal liability rather than protecting the rights of patients.

2. Many committees limit the participation of patients or their family members in decision-making of the committee, and thus the most important components of ethical discipline are left out.

3. Since the committee is loaded with physicians, the mediations and recommendations may reflect the values of the medical profession rather than the values of the patient.

4. The tendency of some committees to operate in secrecy, to omit recommendations in the medical record, or refusing to permit

review of their recommendations, castes certain doubts on the integrity of those committees.

In order to overcome these lapses, the following three points may be considered:

1. From an ethical point of view, it seems clear that the HEC is not a surrogate, and so it is not authorized to make decisions for incompetent patients or their surrogates. Only the law can give such authorization.
2. Even though the HEC is not a surrogate, when consulting on ongoing cases, the ethics committee can and should act primarily as a guardian of patient's rights.
3. The functions of the committee should be clearly and publicly announced, and its recommendations and decisions should be kept open to review.

Summary:

Ethics has been described as the science of morals or rules of conduct concerning human life. Several ethical theories have been postulated by philosophers, which are useful to the people to lead a morally good life and to resolve moral conflicts in their day to day life. Professional ethics is a form of applied ethics, and it promulgates a code of conduct to the members of a particular profession. Medical ethics deals with the principles and values appropriate to the persons working in the area of medical practice.

The roles assigned to health care professionals change from society to society and from time to time as they are influenced by value systems of a given society and goals of the profession. The primary ethical object for the people in medical profession should be to protect the dignity and autonomy of the patients and they should take the informed consent of the patients before they start the treatment.

Further, the principle of beneficence asserts "doing good" to every individual and the principle of nonmaleficence requires "avoiding evil" to all persons. Thus these two principles directly refer to the Hippocrates oath, which is obligatory to every genuine medical practitioner.

Human beings have an intrinsic worth or dignity which makes them valuable above all other things. The Golden Rule Principle says: "treat others only in ways that you would be willing to be treated yourself". We must always recognize and respect humanity in others. Therefore, humans should not be used as means to an end. The demands of human dignity are crucial in medical ethics. The principles of truthfulness and confidentiality must be properly balanced while dealing with the patients by the physicians.

In recent times, the physician patient relationship as a personal and professional relationship is changed due to the advent of corporate hospitals, where the physician works as a businessman and the hospital functions as a business firm with serious consequences for the patient, health care system, and health care ethics. Unless a regulatory body concentrates on this 'corporate culture' the health of a common man is in danger.

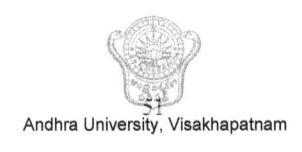

References:

1. Y.V. Satyanarayana, *"Ethics: Theory and Practice"*. (Delhi, Pearson Education, 2010) P.3.

2. Cf. J.S.Mill, *"Utilitarianism"* (Indianapolis, Bobbs–Merrill, 1957), pp.14-18.

3. Cf. Immanuel Kant, *"Foundations of the Metaphysics of Morals"*, translated by L.W.Beck, (New York, Bobbs – Merril, 1959), pp.10-12.

4. Aristotle, *"Nicomachean Ethics"*, translated by W.D.Ross (Oxford, Oxford University Press, 1915), pp.1103a, 1103b.

5. Y.V.Satyanarayana, *"Ethics: Theory and Practice"*, (Delhi, Pearson, 2010), p.47.

6. Jacques P. Thiroux, *"Ethics: Theory and Practice"*, (California, Glexoe Publishing Co., INC., 1977), pp.265-267.

7. Cf. J.A. Rosoff, *"Informed Consent: A Guide for Health Care Providers"* (Rockville, Md; Apsen, 1981), p.14.

8. A.F.Rosovsky, *"Consent to Treatment, A practical Guide"* (Boston, Brown, Little and Co., 1984), pp.98-102.

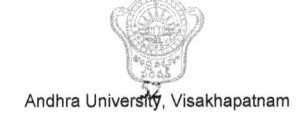

@@@@@

Chapter Three

Ethical Issues Involved in HIV/AIDS Screening

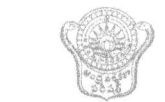

CHAPTER - III

ETHICAL ISSUES INVOLVED IN HIV/ AIDS SCREENING

The four letters word AIDS has been shaking the world since its very inception at the United States of America. Almost every nation has been reporting cases of AIDS to the World Health Organization (WHO), an agency of the United Nations that monitors the AIDS epidemic.

History:

In 1981, the first few cases of AIDS (Acquired Immune Deficiency Syndrome) were identified among gay men in the United States, acquiring the designation GRID (Gay Related Immune Deficiency). However, scientists later found evidence that the disease existed in the world for some years prior to 1981, and subsequent analysis of a blood sample of a Bantu man, who died of an unidentified illness in the Belgian Congo in 1959 made him the first confirmed case of an HIV infection.

In an article, "Where did HIV (Human Immuno Deficiency Virus) come from?", Wain Hobson wrote that both the AIDS viruses, HIV-1 and HIV-2 were originated in Africa".[1]

It has been an ongoing debate about the origin and spread of AIDS. Scientists are not certain how, when, and where the AIDS viruses evolved and first infected humans. Researches have shown that HIV- and HIV-2 are more closely related to Simian Immune Deficiency viruses which infect monkeys. Thus, it has been suggested that HIV evolved from viruses which originally infected monkeys in Africa and was somehow it is transmitted to people.[2]

A Century History of AIDS Virus:

The AIDS virus previously thought to have been transmitted from Chimpanzees to human beings. In October 2008 scientists announced that almost a century ago in the 1930s, in West-Central Africa the virus might have leapt the species barrier. Analysis of tissues preserved by doctors in the colonial-era Belgian Congo showed that the most pervasive strain of the human immunodeficiency virus (HIV) began spreading among humans at some point between 1884 and 1924. "The diversification of HIV-1 in West-Central Africa occurred long before the recognition of AIDS pandemic", they announced in the British- based journal "Nature".

Acquired Immune Deficiency Syndrome first came to public notice in 1981, when the US doctors alerted and noticed an unusual cluster of deaths among young homosexuals in California and New York. Since then, it killed at least 25 million people, and about 33 million others are living with the disease HIV, the virus that causes AIDS by destroying immune cells.

HIV is a highly mutating virus with as much as 1% of its genome diverging per year. As such HIV deviates from previous strains and from its animal ancestor the simian immunodeficiency virus (SIV). By this calculation, HIV might began to spread among humans before 1940.[3]

Scientists believe that HIV infection became widespread after significant social changes took place in Africa during the 1960's and 1970's. Large number of people moved from rural areas to cities, resulting in crowding, unemployment and prostitution. These conditions brought about an increase in cases of sexually transmitted diseases including AIDS. HIV might have been introduced into industrial nations several times before transmission was sustained and became widespread.

When AIDS was first identified as a "new" disease by doctors in Los Angels and New York City in 1980 and 1981, the doctors recognized the condition as something new because all the patients who were previously healthy, young homosexual men suffering from otherwise rare forms of cancer and pneumonia. The name AIDS was adopted in 1982. Scientists soon have come to the conclusion that AIDS is the outcome of HIV infection to a person, and it damages the immune systems of that person, and it spreads from the infected person to others through sexual contact, shared drug needles, or infected blood transfusions.

After HIV was identified as the cause of AIDS in 1983 and 1984, researchers developed tests to detect HIV infection. These tests have been used to analyse the stored tissues from several people who died of undetermined causes in the 1960's and 1970's. On the basis of results of these tests, the scientists have come to the conclusion that some of these people died of AIDS.

Nobel Prize for Virus Discoveries:

Luc Montagnier, director of the World Foundation for AIDS research and prevention, and Francoise Barre-Sinoussi of the Institute of Pasteur have won half the prize of 10 million Swedish Crowns ($1.4 million) for discovering the deadly virus that has killed millions of people since it gained notoriety in the 1980s.These two French scientists identified virus production in lymphocytes from patients in the early stages of acquired immunodeficiency and in blood from patients with late stages of the diseases. The virus became known as human immunodeficiency virus or HIV.[4]

Luc Montagnier has dedicated his award to AIDS sufferers, and predicted results on a "therapeutic vaccine" for the pandemic within four years i.e., by the end of 2012, provided sufficient financial support is given to his team. "I think I did my share", said Barre-Sinoussi. The winner wants more money in AIDS research and flow of new ideas, especially in the field of vaccines, which is "a failure so far".[5]

Several arguments came at this stage about the origin of AIDS. In Africa, certain tribes eat the meat of green monkeys and apply the blood of monkeys on genetalia as an aphrodisiac. During the process of capturing the monkeys, men might have been bitten or scratched by them and hence the SIV (Simian Immuno Deficiency Virus) that remained in the monkeys might have been transferred to humans. In humans, by mutation, the SIV might have been transformed into HIV.

The other argument was that, the Scientists in New York labs while developing a biological war weapon created a new virus, which by accident might have spread into the personnel working in the lab and their contact to others and so on.

Saddam Hussain was blamed for producing and storing the biological war weapons. This might be one of the principal reasons for his death penalty by hanging. The biological war weapon might be developed with Anthrax or HIV, who knows it?

In addition to these arguments, several racial, social, and ethical controversies have been emerging in every corner of the globe. One journalist aptly commented to the theory of origin of HIV in Africa and said that this world is so mischievous that if anything good happens, the credit is attributed to the West, and if anything bad happens the blame is thrown on Africa.

The origin and spread of AIDS the misconceptions and rumors about AIDS, the superstitions roaming around AIDS, and the phobia of AIDS – all these facets have raised several moral dilemmas and conflicts, and a myriad of ethical arguments on what is right and what is wrong, which is negative, and which is positive and causing many confusing viewpoints.

Andhra University, Visakhapatnam

Ethics of HIV/AIDS Screening — Some Misconceptions:

Since 1981, the very first few cases of AIDS identified in the USA, and the horror created by media about AIDS patients, resulted in the lack of interest by general public to go for HIV screening voluntarily, though the HIV tests were readily available in private and public sector health care institutions.

HIV testing outside the context of blood transfusion and blood banking requires consideration of several ethical issues, which includes informed consent, confidentiality, voluntary counseling and testing, etc., and these factors must be ensured so that more and more people with high risk behaviour, and the general public would come forward to undergo HIV testing to help themselves and the community.

Testing and Screening:

HIV testing or screening of persons or populations has been challenged in a wide variety of settings, including the judiciary, corrections system, health care, public health, insurance and employment. Testing or screening programmes have been challenged under several legal suits. In India, general screening for HIV was offered at many voluntary counseling and testing centers under national AIDS control organization. HIV testing involves issues of privacy, communal health, social and economic discrimination, coercion and liberty. HIV testing evoked huge controversy and debate, involving matters, such as should all the individuals with high risk are to be tested? How and who will counsel those in case they turn to be positive? What about confidentiality? What about the consequences of testing, with regard to one's right to work, to go to school, to get married, to bear children and to obtain insurance? These types of emerging issues have different ethical bearings in their day to day life. It is so difficult to imagine the upcoming intrinsic moral dilemmas. Except for clearly restricted circumstance, HIV testing has to be performed under conditions of voluntary informed consent and the results are to be protected by stringent confidentiality safe guards.

HIV screening /testing can be undertaken as voluntary testing after counseling for behaviour change; for clinical purposes, for seroprevalence studies; for ensuring safety and for research. There is lot of debate on routine mandatory testing.

Those who support routine mandatory testing argue that the infected persons can be identified early and counseled about HIV/AIDS. Secondly, patients can be treated sooner to prevent progression of disease and limit complications. Thirdly, it benefits the health care workers so that they can take special care to protect themselves from accidental exposure while treating known HIV infected patients.

The opponents of mandatory testing argue that testing large number of people is not cost effective and is rather counter productive. The voluntary screening after counseling is more effective and productive for behaviour change and case management. For health care workers, practice of standard work precautions will be more beneficial in the light of window period and other blood transmitted infections like hepatitis B and C.[6]

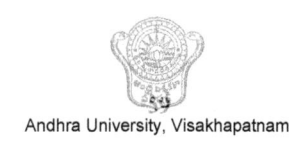

Widely available HIV testing facilities in private and government institutions allowed many people to go for testing of their status. In the past there was a custom of pre-test counseling and post-test counseling. However, the lacuna in the system and the poor and unsuccessful counseling resulted in several suicides of the positive people. For example, a young engineering student, after seeing his test report collected from voluntary counseling and testing center hanged himself in a hotel room with a suicide note that he got a dreadful disease, and he may be ill treated by the people around him and his life may be miserable in the society.

This shows the perceptions of a common man about the test results of HIV. It is a very sensitive issue, and what right do the testing centers have to promote suicides of innocent youth due to lack of proper skills in counseling at their end? If mass screening is advocated without due care of the mindset of the people, there is no wonder to imagine that the place in the existing graveyards may not be sufficient for the future catastrophes. Hence, mass screening of HIV is definitely unethical, because it may lead to a large number of suicides. Nevertheless mass screening can be adopted when majority people realize or treat HIV/ AIDS as another manageable chronic disease and avoid subjecting them for suicides. In India, many hospitals have been conducting mandatory HIV testing of the pregnant women who go for antenatal checkup. Well, this procedure is initiated to identify the positive status of woman and to administer the ART drug to prevent mother to child transmission. Here also due to poor confidentiality measures of HIV test results major mishaps are happening.

In 2007, in Guntur district of Andhra Pradesh (India), after knowing the test result of his wife as positive, a young man brutally killed his wife and he himself committed suicide. And in another case in the State of Bihar, a seven months pregnant mother of two children having known her status of HIV positive at an antenatal check up center, died by taking poison along with her two children. These episodes have a clear message that how grave the HIV positive news and its consequences leading to killings and suicides. Here I would like to raise a question, what ethical considerations are being thought of by organizing mandatory testing at antenatal check up centers. Is it legitimate to continue the same system without providing adequate safeguard of proper counseling to the innocent pregnant women? The screening of HIV may be beneficial to a large section of population, but suicides and killings have high moral burden on the society. Social issues are related to ethical issues. Contrary to empowering women in society, creating circumstances for humiliation and provoking suicides is a curse to the society. AIDS, in its every stage is shaking the cultural norms, social values and the humane principles.

Due to weak administration, the HIV status is being leaked out and it is interfering with the peaceful and respectful living of those women who have undergone mandatory tests at the antenatal centers. Is it not a form of violation of human rights to reveal confidential matters to others? But the testing centers argue that they are doing group counseling and individual counseling as and where it is essential, but it looks as though the system they are following is not praiseworthy.

Laboratory testing for HIV infection is the definite way to detect infection even in the persons who looks healthy, who are other wise called as asymptomatic carriers. A number of ethical, legal and psycho-social issues are related to HIV testing. HIV/AIDS is a complex and unique infectious disease. The infection is life long and as on today no successful cure or vaccine is available. Hence, anyone attempting to assess the HIV status of a person, must be convergent with the issues and related strategies of testing, protocols of testing, rationale of using particular test, correct method of informing the result to the client, importance of counseling, maintaining confidentiality, technical and other pit falls, and practice of quality assurance.

National AIDS control organization (NACO) has developed the national policy on HIV testing as a part of the National AIDS control programme.

False Positive or False Negative HIV Test Results:

Due to several factors, a person may be given either false positive or false negative results. Both these results can create enough ambiguity in the clients. Nevertheless, the false positive test result, without actual infection, may create disastrous consequences to the persons concerned and they may commit suicides. Socially and psychologically, HIV test by itself is very sensitive and even the slightest mistake by technician or data entry operator or the lapse material used can explode myriad problems. Similarly, the false negative test result may make a person more comfortable transiently and one may be complacent and may contribute for spreading of HIV silently to the innocent people, may be to his/her partner or spouse.

Both false positive and false negative results may also occur due to errors committed by the technologists, and due to use of expired kits or reagents.[7] There is also possibility of contamination of samples and wrong labeling can result in havoc of test results.

Human life is at risk due to the false positive and false negative HIV results. People who are more emotional, more sensitive and more anxious and fickle minded may take undesirable decisions in a fraction of a minute due to wrong test results. Human life is sacred and invaluable, and it loses its significance in the wake of HIV inaccurate test results.

Testing in Error:

GMC (General Medical Council) guidance states that mistakes should be acknowledged, with apology and appropriate support offered. The patient must be given the choice as to whether they are given the result of the test. If the patient refuses to receive a positive result (with health implications for that individual, partners, and others) then advice should be obtained from professional bodies. In the Indian context, there is an immediate need to evolve suitable guidelines for smoothening and relief to the victims in case of errors in testing for HIV.

Epidemiological Studies:

Testing for epidemiological purposes (e.g. for HIV, Hepatitis C virus) is important for planning disease management, but it raises some ethical issues. It generally involves screening surplus material (e.g. serum) taken for other tests to allow meaningful epidemiological data to be obtained ensuring that it cannot be linked to the anonymous individual. However, it is acknowledged that the information gained will not directly benefit that person. It is generally agreed that the benefit to public health outweighs the ethical dilemma of testing without consent to avoid biased sampling. Written information should be available to patients explaining the nature of this testing within the clinic as leaflets or posters which must highlight the option to refuse without prejudice.[8]

In screening tests, the genetic bottleneck is also a subject of discussion. When a study appeared in science suggesting that the virus that establishes HIV infection goes through a severe genetic bottleneck and might be more sensitive to antibody neutralization, it causes quite a stir. Eric Hunter, a professor at Emory University and his colleagues including Derdeyn, studied eight heterosexual transmission pairs from a discordant couple cohort in Zambia, four male-to-females (M-F) and four female-to-males (F-M) subtype C HIV transmission. Viral env sequences, specifically the regional spanning the V1-V4 loops, were studied from peripheral blood mono nuclear cells (PBMCs) and plasma. They found that an external bottleneck occurred in all the transmission, which they interpreted as the transmission or outgrowth of a single sequence from the donor quasispecies.[9]

This diversity of infection of discordant couple where wife is positive, husband is negative and vice versa creating challenging ethical problems and unsolved misunderstandings among the couples. This leads further research as what factors are influencing and what genetic variation is playing a significant role in preventing the transmissions of HIV in discordant couples.

Ethical Problems of Mass Screening:

In mass screening, a large numbers of people, including healthy people, are tested in order to detect a few people. Many might have encountered mass screenings at big shopping malls or hospitals. Everyone is invited here to have their blood sugar checkup or blood pressure check up or tests for TB detection etc. There are two sets of problems connected with mass screening. The first one is an extension of the problems of routine testing. The second one is concerned with the problems of confidentiality and the social stigma attached to it.

Generally, mass screening with asymptomatic population often produce higher rates of false positives. Secondly, when there is no truly effective treatment for the ailments detected, the tests may be useless. The AIDS testing illustrates both the points. The consequences of either false positive or false negative can be extremely serious. The false negative gives false security and leaves the illness untreated. The false positive can torture patients and expose them to unnecessary and even dangerous treatments. Sometimes, as in the case of HIV/AIDS, the false positive is an apparent death sentence that can lead to both despair and suicide. If the test results are not kept confidential, they could also lead to isolation, discrimination, social stigma, and loss of employment. Both types of error can also expose the doctor/health care professional to make practice suits.[10]

Therefore, voluntary screening may be ethical if the person is told who will have access to the results and what harmful consequences may result. The voluntary screenings of people by government organizations need justification in terms of the public good. In either screening, the danger of stigmatization, the high cost of drugs and the dangers to confidentiality need special consideration.

The HIV screening or the HIV test, though it is simple to perform, its results have tremendous significance for both individuals and the communities where they live. Hence, it has been an ongoing controversy on HIV test. In the beginning, HIV tests were performed on high risk group individuals such as long distance lorry drivers, intravenous (IV) drug users, sex workers, but later the test is offered to each and every individual with a pre-test and post-test counseling. However, it has been mandatory at antenatal clinics in India after group pretest counseling. Recently CDC, Atlanta suggested to have HIV test whenever indicated by the treating physician without any pre-test counseling. Mr. Obama, the President of USA would like to introduce HIV testing for general public, and he suggested that everyone should have voluntarily the HIV test so that the prevention of HIV would be more successful.

In India, NACO started "Be Bold" campaign with a message... "That who ever are bold can come forward for HIV testing." In the 2nd week of July, 2009, the Government of Andhra Pradesh has initiated a programme namely *"Shubham"*, with a call to the people of Andhra Pradesh, "Let us come forward for the screening of HIV/AIDS", and let us detect the danger in advance. Whatever be the name given for HIV screening, the fears in the minds of common man about the profound stigma is always haunting him. Unless the civil societies, the governments, the NGOs, and the religious leaders belonging to all major religions, strive to create an unstigmatized environment in the society, AIDS free world will be a day dream.

The issues posed by the HIV test may change as the therapeutic context changes. But what cannot change is the enduring necessity of careful analysis of the ethical and social implications of policies designed to guide the use of the test. The testing policies compel us to consider matters of privacy, dignity and social welfare. As such, they enforce us to confront the most significant questions of ethical issues and human rights provoked by HIV/AIDS.

Screening for Clinical Purposes:

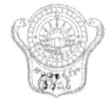

Early in the history of the epidemic, the question with which some patients and many of their advocates confronted those who proposed antibody testing was, "of what benefit will a positive finding be for me?" Furthermore, this was not a test like any other typically employed by clinicians.

It is not a malaria, typhoid or dengue fever test to readily accept, rather, it was argued, the antibody test was for social and psychological reasons more like those invasive procedures for which special consent was required. Faced with such challenges, and the undeniable reality of social stigma associated with HIV infection, physicians, their professional associations and public health officials agreed that an exact standard of consent, for HIV testing and an appropriate informed consent is to be sought from patients or their surrogates. However, to many clinicians such requirements are resulting in unhealthy relationship with the patients.[11]

HIV Testing in Pregnancy:

In 1985, The Centers for Disease Control and Prevention (CDC) USA recommended that medical providers discourage women known to be HIV positive from child bearing as a mechanism for preventing prenatal HIV transmission. In 1987, CDC recommended prenatal HIV antibody testing for all pregnant women at risk for HIV infection. In 1994 and 1995, the CDC issued recommendations regarding HIV counseling, voluntary testing and use of Zidovudine (ZDV) to prevent prenatal transmission of HIV. The working group on HIV testing observed that screening of all pregnant women should be informed about HIV transmission, and offered counseling and voluntary testing. This can be counted as most reasonable and effective approach.[12]

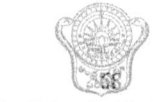

This option seems to be most suited for India also, but we need to have more trained counselors to follow this procedure. Ideally, all pregnant women should be given informed choice about HIV testing.

In Early 1980s, many pregnant women were forcibly convinced to go for abortion to prevent vertical transmission of HIV. With inadequate knowledge on the rates of transmission of HIV from mother to child, brutal killings of fetuses left irreparable wounds in the wombs of mothers. They used to cry silently. Their tears, their agony, and their dumbness for their failure to beget a child cannot be expressed in words. It's beyond ones imagination. One may argue that it is justifiable as we have no right to allow a positive child born on the earth to suffer all humiliations, recurrent infections, stigma discrimination, and premature death. The other argument is that not all children born to HIV positive mothers are getting infection and even without any intervention or treatment to prevent mother to child transmission about 55% negative children are born. Then how far is it ethical to destroy the motherliness of women as well as the fetuses. Still it is an ongoing debate. In spite of the modern ART drugs that are available to significantly reduce HIV transmission from mother to child, the moral dilemmas continue to prevail.

There are still shameful occurrences of efforts to exclude or isolate school children with AIDS or HIV infection. Many cases of discrimination by employers continue to occur, and such discrimination is almost universally deplored as irrational, unscientific and ethically unacceptable. Thus, in the United States, the CDC centers for disease control moved swiftly to contain the irrational impulse towards exclusion. So at the end of 1985, separate guidelines were issued to prevent the spread of HIV infection in schools and the workplaces.[13] In early 1986 the detailed guidelines on preventing the spread of infection when health care workers are engaged in invasive procedure were published.[14]

In each of these instances, the goal is to convey information, to provide protection, and to prevent panic. The message is very clear that HIV could not be casually transmitted, and so there is no reason for exclusion from school and workplace of infected individuals who were otherwise capable of performing their expected functions. In the context of the health care setting, universal blood and body fluid precautions would protect workers not only from HIV but also from the far more infections such as hepatitis B. Screening would only provide illusory protections.

HIV and Pregnancy:

HIV infection does not reduce a woman's desire and hopes for sexual bonding, intimacy, and child bearing. The rise in prevalence of HIV among women attending antenatal clinics is a point for concern as this is an indicator of disease in general population. Also the rise in number of HIV infected children indicates the rise of infection in women of child bearing age group.

In India, the HIV epidemic is quite heterogeneous in distribution and prevalence of HIV in antenatal women varies widely. The sentinel surveillance data from antenatal clinics in 7 metro cities in the country shows that HIV infection has crossed 2% in Mumbai; it is over 1% in Hyderabad, Bangalore and Chennai and is below 1% in Kolkata, Ahmadabad and Delhi.

Measures to Prevent Vertical Transmission:

All HIV infected pregnant women should be given an informed choice about medical termination of pregnancy (MTP). If the woman chooses it, safe MTP services should be provided to her. If she decides to continue with pregnancy, she should be told about risk of child getting infected and the role of antiretroviral therapy especially ZDV in reducing this risk. All pregnant women should be offered ZDV therapy. The ante-partum care should be tailored to these specific needs with ample psychosocial support. In the ante-partum period, close monitoring of CD4 cell counts should be done and appropriate prophylaxis for various infections should be used as and when required.

HIV Testing before Marriage:

In the light of a considerable number of young boys and girls are being HIV positive, a great debate is going on whether to make HIV testing compulsory before marriage or not. One argument is that it should not be made mandatory at the instance of family members. This will erode the voluntary component of the VCTC (Voluntary Confidential Counseling and Testing). Further this may lead to the victimization of individuals found to be HIV positive. It must be ensured that young people, who request premarital HIV testing, do so voluntarily and not under pressure from the family, clergy etc., and many governments such as Andhra Pradesh, Orissa, Gujarat, have initiated the process of enactment of law on this issue. Marriage is a sacred bondage, an embodiment of trust between man and woman, and a socially respectful event, which is surrounded by sentiments of different cultures. It is a very sensitive matter where intrusion of HIV testing before marriage may open up several legal, moral, social and cultural problems. At the same time, in the wake of about 0.8 – 1% of incidence of HIV among adolescents in India, blindly performing marriages without checking HIV status of bride and bridegroom may end in a catastrophe if one of the couple turns positive.

The following incident which happened in recent times illustrates the seriousness of the HIV problem for Young boys and girls who decided to marry.

In November 2007, on a snowfall day, around 5 am a middle aged man came to my residence and rang the calling bell. That day happens to be Sunday, I was little lazy to respond to the bell, but I could not be silent for his long calling bell second time. When I came out and saw him, he was in deep anguish, and before I asked him what the matter is, he said: "Sir, by what time you come to the clinic? Today my daughter's marriage is fixed at 9:45 pm. Last night someone called me on phone and told me that my would-be son-in-law had AIDS. On hearing this news, I and my wife were very much shocked. So far, we have not revealed this matter either to my daughter or any other family member. We are in a fix whether to go ahead with the marriage or cancel it. We have also invited about 500 people for a marriage feast this afternoon. Meanwhile, my wife advised me to contact you to verify the HIV status of my would-be son in law. I could not sleep the whole night. I'm sorry to disturb you so early in the morning."

After listening to him, I was thinking for a short while, and I sympathized with his plight of affair where he stands in a critical situation between his daughter's marriage and son-in-law's HIV status. I told him to come to my clinic immediately with his would be son-in-law, though I usually don't go so early on Sundays to the clinic, which is nearly 6 kms away from my residence.

Around 6 A.M., I performed quick antibody test on his blood sample and to all of our grief surprise, the report came positive. The bride's parents collapsed in front of me in my clinic. With great difficulty, my staff and I could reconcile them. However, they broke out loudly imagining the difficult situation they have to face with their relatives, friends, and all other people who are invited to attend for the lunch and the other marriage related events on that day. They pleaded me to give my opinion whether to stop the marriage at this juncture or not. I kept silent without giving my opinion to them. One can imagine what would be the mental state of these innocent parents of the bride having spent lot of money, paid dowry in advance, and distributed all wedding invitations. Dreadfully few hours before the wedlock, this news about their would-be son-in-law falls on them like a thunder stroke.

Though I suspected in the beginning that it may be a foul play of some rival of the bridegroom to spoil the marriage by spreading such rumors, but the result of the test turned to be positive is a great shocking news. This incident, despite a tragedy to the pre-marital bride, HIV testing could save the life of the tender girl. Disease like HIV/AIDS, with no complete cure or potent vaccine, is almost a death warrant with a horrifying social stigma attached to it, should not be allowed to transmit silently in a memorable event of life like marriage.

No parents want their daughter or son to become chronically ill or sick on bed or die prematurely. The dreadful HIV is not only causing an irreparable damage to a trusted bondage but also erasing fundamental fabrics of marriage system. It is opening Pandora box and posing a number of questions about the very nature of ethics of marriage. If the bride or the bridegroom knowingly and intentionally conceals their positive status of HIV virus, and prepare for the marriage, then it is a big blow to the values that are associated with the institution of marriage.

In this context, Legal experts, ethicists, and holy persons should have a brainstorm session to find out a universally acceptable solution, without hurting the fond feelings and gentle hearts of the couples. However, as a physician and social activist, I would support the premarital HIV tests on a consensual basis for both prospective bride and bridegroom in the best interest of the couple as well as in the interest of yet to be born children to them.

It is better if both bride and bridegroom voluntarily come forward for HIV testing, irrespective of mandatory HIV testing or Government's enactment of law in this matter. Nevertheless, one must be cautions when performing HIV tests on prospective couples, in view of false positive and false negative test results. In a country like India, where many labs are not nationally accredited, there is a possibility of issuing spurious or false results of HIV tests by some unethical lab personnel. Further, unless we come out with highly advanced tests like nucleic acid tests or repeated polymerase chain reaction (PCR) tests to detect HIV in window period, a massive danger of wrong test results is lurking around. The conventional, widely used antibody HIV tests cannot detect the incidence of HIV in window period. A window period is that period which is required to produce sufficient antibodies for the virus. A person carrying HIV may give negative test result in window period, with the routinely performed antibody test. But he/she is still infectious and can transmit the virus potently. If anyone considers the negative test in window period, may be direct victim of the HIV infection.[15]

Society has for long accepted the desirability of VDRL testing as a prerequisite for marriage. There is no reason why the same cannot be done with HIV testing which remains the only protection for the young Indian men and women and their unborn children.

Poverty, powerlessness, and social instability promote the spread of both HIV and other STIs. Due to lack of employment many people are forced to migrate to the urban areas where a high incidence of HIV/STIs prevails. The impact of an increased HIV/STI on the public health of a community is very serious. The high prevalence of STIs is known to increase HIV transmission. The consequences of HIV/AIDS may lead to social rejection, isolation, loss of income, poverty, and economic dependence. The community has to take responsibility to support an increasing number of orphans born to AIDS couples. Hence it is the need of the hour to bring about social emancipation through increased awareness about human rights and sexual/reproductive health in every section of the population in view of impending risks, which may jeopardize positive people.[16]

Problems of Marriage of HIV Positive People:

HIV positives when they are young, either a positive man or a positive woman would make an effort for a marriage due to several cultural factors and social norms. In some cultures, if the eldest in the family is not married, the next to him is usually not allowed to go for a marriage. In some other situations, if a positive boy or girl in a family is not married when they reach the marriageable age and if their parents won't perform their mirage, the relatives, the friends and the community question them the reasons for the delay, and criticize them if the marriage is overdue. The positive man, for the fear of society or with the sentiment not to spoil the life of other innocent young girl, may prefer to live unmarried throughout his life. Same may be the case with fair sex. In some other special circumstances, due to pressure from parents or family members or friends, some positive young people without intimating their status to the bride or their family may marry the innocent negative girl or healthy girl. These types of marriages are happening day in and day out in between positive boy and negative girl and vice versa, but the latter is considerably low in number. Kant says that using a person as a means to an end is most unethical. In the panoramic view of AIDS, marriages have become very crucial events. Added to this, some positive young men are marrying positive young ladies or positive widows. Some sociologists argue that the marriage is a cultural norm, not only living together but is also a kind of bondage between man and woman.

In case of a marriage between a positive man and a negative girl, without informing the boy's positive status, the role of parents cannot be undermined. The parents want that their son should be married so that they will get social status, but they never bother about the future life of the poor innocent negative girl. We don't understand how the parents are encouraging such unethical practice. If their son is not married, their progeny may be ended may be the apprehension of the parents. This practice is highly unethical because the bride is used as a means to satisfy the aim of bridegroom's parents. Some one may argue that the positive man is having marriage only for the sake of having companionship but not to beget children. This statement looks very sacred but how far it will be genuinely practiced? Some couples may go for barrier methods. The positive couple when they are in psychological depression or in upset mood due to their positive status and related family based, society based repercussions, they still like to go for a marriage publicly or privately with a philosophy that "Marriages are made in Heaven". However this popular saying is loosing its charm in the world of AIDS.

For a HIV positive person, if someone agrees to be a companion with full compassion and deep love, then he/she considers it as a fortune and enjoys it as a heaven. It is not that easy for a HIV positive person to have spouse or a partner or a companion with good understanding. However, one should appreciate the sentiments behind living together any positive couple for that matter their life is worth living when we compare them with those who unethically betrayed the innocent negative girls in the name of marriage.

Summary:

Since 1981 the first few cases of AIDS were identified, till to day AIDS disease has been center of discussion for the policy makers of public health world over. HIV -1 and HIV – 2, the two strains are thought to be evolved from viruses which originally infected monkeys in Africa. Man's association with monkeys might have facilitated the HIV transmission to human beings. Luc Montagnier and Barre Sinoussi got noble award for the discovery of HIV (Human immuno deficiency virus) in 2009.

The mysterious origin and the rapid spread of AIDS, well before the discovery of causative agent have brought forth several phobias and misconceptions about AIDS, which in turn raised many ethical dilemmas in dealing with HIV/AIDS patients.

When we want to test a person for malaria, or for typhoid, usually there is no need of informed consent, confidentiality, and counseling etc, whereas for testing a person for HIV, diverse ethical issues have to be considered. Incase the HIV test results turns to be positive some sensitive individuals are undergoing great psychological trauma and committing suicides or going underground. This situation is a huge stumbling block for effective control of HIV/AIDS.

In recent times, compulsory HIV testing before marriage is an issue for debate. How it is to be implemented without hurting the fond feelings and gentle hearts of the couples is a question. Otherwise, many innocent brides are being infected and few bridegrooms are also getting infected, vice versa. In general, no parent wants his son or daughter to be a chronically ill or sick on bed or die prematurely with AIDS. Both brides and bridegrooms voluntarily come forward for HIV testing in the interest of their health and future offspring. The marriage between positive couples is a positive change in the society. Companionship with mutual love and compassion will infuse new life in them to work towards a better society.

References:

1. Simon Wain. Hobson, "1959 and all that: Immunodeficiency Viruses", in *"Nature"* Volume 391 (United Kingdom, Nature publishing group, 1998). Pp. 532-533

2. 'History of AIDS', *"The World Book Encyclopedia"* (Chicago USA, © World Book Inc. 2005) pp. 181-182.

3. N. Ram (ed), *"The Hindu"* (Chennai, The Hindu, 2008) p. 18

4. N. Ram (ed), *"The Hindu"* (Chennai, The Hindu, 2008) p. 1

5. Aditya Sinha (ed), *"The New Indian Express"* (Chennai, Express Publications Ltd., 2008) p. 4

6. Bayer. R, and Gostin LO. "HIV Screening and Ethical Issues". in Jayasuriya D.C, (ed) *"HIV: Law Ethics and Human Rights"* (New Delhi, UNDP 1995) pp. 295-311

7. Cordes RJ, and Ryan ME. "Pitfalls in HIV Testing: Applications and Limitations of Current Tests" in *"Post grad Med"* (Bethesda, USA, © National Center for biotechnology information 1995) pp.177-180

8. Richard Pattman and Michael Snow (eds), "Ethical and Medico Legal Issues", in *"Oxford Handbook of Genitourinary Medicine, HIV, and AIDS"*, (London, Oxford University Press, 2007) p. 23.

9. Simon Noble, 'HIV Transmission: The Genetic Bottleneck', *"IAVI Report Vol.12, no.6"* (USA, International AIDS vaccine initiative, 2008) P. 5

10. Thomas M. Garrett, Harold W. Baillie and Rosellen M. Garrett "The Ethics of Testing and Screening" in *"Health Care Ethics: Principles and Problems"*, (Switzerland, Pearson Education Schweiz AG, 2007) pp.199-207.

11. Ronald Bayer and Larry O. Gostin, "HIV Screening: The Ethical Issues" in *"HIV Law: Ethics and Human Rights"*, (New Delhi, UNDP, 1995) p.298.

12. Chavkin W, Brietbart V, and Wise P. State *"HIV Maternal Child Health Policies and Programmes"* (Washington DC, HIV infection in women conference, 1995) (Abst. WB 2-37)

13. "CDC Recommendations for preventing transmission of infection with human T-lymphotropic virus type III/lymphedenopathy-

associated virus in the work place" *"MMWR"* (USA, Centers for Disease Control, 1984) V 34: pp. 681-86, 691-95.

14. "Centers for Disease Control: Recommendations for preventing transmission of infection with human T-lymphotropic virus type III/lymphedenopathy-associated virus during invasive procedures" *"MMWR"* (USA, CDC, 1986) V 35, pp. 221-223.

15. RD Lele. "HIV-AIDS", in *"Text Book of Family Medicine"*, (Chennai, I.M.A College of general practitioners, 2005), p. 313.

16. Kutikuppala Surya Rao, et. al., 'Sexual/reproductive health in the wake of HIV/AIDS in relation to human rights- a pilot study'. *"The Antiseptic Vol. 100 No. 9"* (Madurai, Professional Publications Pvt. Ltd., 2003), p. 361.

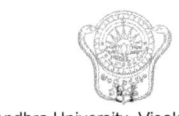

@@@@@

Chapter Four

Legal and Moral issues Relating to AIDS

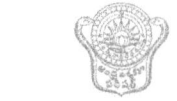

CHAPTER IV

LEGAL AND MORAL ISSUES RELATING TO AIDS

AIDS – Legal Issues:

The Supreme Court of India, recently approved the direction of the Government of India, issued to all states that doctors in government and private hospitals should not refuse treatment to the people living with HIV/AIDS. The Supreme Court Bench consisting of Chief Justice K.G. Balakrishnan, Justice Ashok Bhan, and justice P. Sathasivam observed that all states should implement the instruction of the central government forthwith.

The Government of India order says that "All doctors, nurses and hospital staff, whether in the public or private sector, shall treat people living with HIV/AIDS (PLHA) in a professional manner, and treat them always with dignity and care. No doctor or nurse shall refuse to treat PLHA on account of their HIV positive status. In treating PLHA, there shall be no discrimination of stigma whatsoever".

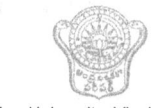

It also states: "Doctors in the private sector, in particular, are directed to immediately familiarize themselves with the National AIDS Control Organisation (NACO) comprehensive protocols and policies with regard to care and treatment. The NACO approved Anti Retroviral Treatment (ART) regimen which has proven to be cost effective, safe and PLHA's have shown good response to this regimen".

Cases of denial of services to positive patients should be viewed seriously, and action to be initiated against those who refuse to treat. The government said, strict action must be taken on all irrational prescriptions of ART. All false advertisements offering potential cure for HIV must be banned, and such individuals and organizations should be dealt with strictly, as there is no proven cure available for HIV/AIDS so far.[1] The instructions issued by the Supreme Court of India, if implemented correctly, will protect the human rights of the AIDS patients and boost up their morale.

Can HIV be the Sole Ground for Discharging a Man from Army?

The Supreme Court examined a case whether a person serving in the army can be discharged on the sole ground of his being HIV positive. The petitioner served the army for 24 years. His HIV positive status was detected during a blood donation camp in 1999. Subsequently, he was given a category called permanent medical classification that is assigned usually to HIV positive persons who are not on ART. In December 2007, Mr. Ved Prakash was put on ART and the medical officer certified that he was capable of performing the duties. He was promoted from the Naik to the Havaldar rank. However subsequently, he was discharged from service. The Delhi high court granted the interim stay against his discharge from service but later vacated it. In his special leave petition, against the high court order, Ved Prakash said that under the guidelines for management and prevention of HIV/AIDS infection in the armed forces, a person might be boarded out only when he shows unsatisfactory response to therapy. But none of the conditions applied in this case.[2] The above case raises the following legal and moral questions:

1. Could an individual be discharged on the erroneous assumption that HIV positive persons were inherently incapable of serving the army?
2. Could the petitioner be discharged erroneously assigning him a medical classification against the guidelines and policy of the government?
3. Does a person be discharged without an order from the medical board invalidating him?

Many Government and private institutions inhumanly started removing several healthy positive persons from service, and throwing them on to the roads miserably. It amounts to violation of a person's right to employment that would result in an unexpected damage to the dependant family members of the victim. Due to sudden loss of employment, his friends and relatives may enquire about the reasons for the loss of job, and it may result in stigma and discrimination. There are also some reported incidents of suicides in such cases. From the viewpoint of the employer, continuing the positive person in the organization may damage its reputation, or he may infect others in the work place, which is only an imaginary assumption that is far from truth. However, the loss of employment causes a great injustice to the healthy and competent positive people, whose sustenance has been simply denied.

Discrimination of HIV positives at work place is the real problem. Most of the private companies do mandatory testing for HIV at the time of employment, and those who are found infected are denied jobs, though the reasons cited are different altogether.

The people who are denied jobs on the basis of HIV discrimination are unwilling to seek legal remedy, fearing wide publicity of their positive status. But the recent judgment passed by the Karnataka Administrative Tribunal is a shot in the arm for those who are willing to seek legal help. The Tribunal has directed the Karnataka State Government to provide job to Mr. R. Ramesh Rao of Shimoga, who was denied a police constable's post due to his HIV positive status in 1999, and the tribunal also ordered that he should be given the job with retrospective effect. The tribunal further directed the State government to ensure that HIV infected people should not be denied government jobs due to their positive status.[3] Many HIV positive people are unaware of these judgments and legal rights they have and hence suffering silently.

Homosexuality and Law:

India took a giant, although a belated step towards globalization when the Delhi High Court delivered a historic judgment to amend a

149 years old British colonial law. On July 2, 2009 the Court struck down the provision of Section 377 of the Indian Penal Code, which criminalised consensual sexual acts of adults in private, holding that it violates the fundamental right of life and liberty, and the right to equality as guaranteed in the Constitution. It is the biggest victory for gay rights, and a major milestone in the country's social evolution. India became the twelfth country to take out the guilt of homosexuality.[3]

A Division Bench consisting of Justice A.P. Shah and Justice S. Muralidhar in its 105-page order said: "We declare that Section 377 of the IPC, insofar as it criminalises consensual sexual acts of adults in private, is violative of article 21 [Right to Protection of Life and Personal Liberty], article 14 [Right to Equality before Law] and article 15 [Prohibition of Discrimination on Grounds of Religion, Race, Caste, Sex or Place of birth] of the Constitution.

The section 377 of India penal code imposes maximum penalty of life sentence on anybody who has "carnal intercourse against the order of nature" with any man, woman or animal.

Upholding the petition filed by NAZ Foundation., the court ruled. 'Indian constitutional law does not permit the statutory criminal law to be held captive by the popular misconceptions about the LGBTs (Lesbian, Gays, Bisexuals and Transgender) people. It cannot be forgotten that discrimination is antithesis of equality, and so it is the recognition of equality which will foster the dignity of every individual."[4]

"There is almost unanimous medical and psychiatric opinion that homosexuality is just another expression of human sexuality", the court said. The verdict triggered protests from religious leaders across the spectrum who invoked the "will of God" to claim the ruling would lead to the "downfall" of society and family values. Political parties were divided on court's verdict; some parties welcome the judgment, while others opposed it.

When Justice Shah pronounced the verdict, a large number of gay activists in the court erupted in celebrations. Many thumped the desk and hugged each other with their eyes filled up with tears. "Now it seems we are in 21st century and the rights of homosexuals have been recognized by the court. This is very progressive judgment, which recognizes the right to equality of homosexuals." The main benefit of the judgment to homosexuals is psychological as it reduces scope for their harassment. There are hardly any instances of section 377 being used against consensual sex between adults, and in course of time, it may reduce the social stigma attached to homosexuality.

The Government is unlikely to appeal unless forced to do so. If someone else goes in appeal, Government will be called upon to take a stand. There are conflicting views whether this verdict apply only to Delhi or to the entire country. The Supreme Court Judgment delivered in 2004 supports the latter view.[5]

The Court Order will Help in HIV Battle:

NACO estimates that 7 out of every 100 men having sex with men have AIDS, and the prevalence of infection within this community is

7.41%. Prejudice against homosexuality is seriously affecting India's fight against the deadly HIV, but the judgment of the Delhi high court promises to be a boon for the country's National AIDS control organisation. Experts says that oppressive laws such as section 377 had driven men who have sex with men (MSM) to underground, making it much harder to reach them with HIV prevention, treatment and care services. India, therefore, is seeing an alarming increase in HIV infection among MSMs.

According to a resent study it has come into light that India is a home for 2.35million MSMs, out of which 100,000 are at high risk of contracting HIV. Already, 15% of this community is infected due to poor access to information and condoms. In this context Dr. Charles Gilks from UNAIDS said, "Section 377 of the IPC, that made homosexuality a criminal offence, was an impediment to our working effectively with the MSM community. Fear of harassment made them to stay away from the public life, thereby making it difficult for us to map the size of this community". Dr. Gilks further added: "It will take a long time to change the public attitude towards MSMs. But this judgment will make it easier for us to reach out to the MSM population and include them in the targeted interventions that will protect them against HIV." However, in several countries, sexual activity between males is punishable by death.[6]

Under India's National AIDS Control Programme II (NACPII), till a year back, only 30 TIs (Targeted interventions) were dealing with the MSM community. The interventions include behavioural change, education, services to treat sexually transmitted infections, providing condoms and lubricants, linking them with integrated counseling and testing centers, and providing them with life saving anti-retroviral drugs if infected. At present, the number of such MSM specific interventions stands at 184, covers 70% of the population. For each TI an amount of Rs 12-18 lakhs per year is allocated for implementation of the programme. Around 30 more TIs are being planned for MSMs and the judgment will help more MSMs to come out in the near future.

Former Health Minister Mr. A. Ram doss, the first person who is in favour of an amendment to section 377, told that now we can reach the MSM community to protect them against HIV. According to government estimates, 5% of all sexually active males in India have sex with other men. A Report from American Foundation for AIDS Research recently said MSMs were 19 times more likely to be infected with HIV than the general population, yet they were ignored in many countries.

Historical Accept of Gay Kiss:

Four thousand years back the first recorded gay kiss or same sex kiss was alleged to depict as a wall painting on a joint tomb of ancient Egyptians. The royal servants namely Khnumhotep and Niankhakhnum, nothing was known about their relationship, but two of the paintings show them with their noses touching each which was the most intimate embrace permitted in Egyptian art of the time used to depict kissing.

French Revolution:

Apart from bringing liberty, equality, and fraternity, the French Revolution also contributed for the abolition of religious courts, which considered sodomy as serious crime punishable with death penalty. The subsequent penal code of 1791 made no mention of sexual relations of consenting adults beyond 21 years age, and France becomes first country of the modern world to decriminalize homosexuality.

Colonial Legacy:

Homosexuality was first mentioned in FLETA, a Treatise on the common law of England, written in 1290. The first law penalizing sodomy was buggery ACT of 1533, reenacted in 1563 by Queen Elizabeth-I. It made sodomy illegal not only in Britain but also in its colonies; The Indian penal code (IPC) was drafted by Lord Macaulay, and it came in force in 1861. It mentions sodomy in the chapter of offences affecting the human body.

Gay Sex Unnatural:

The Delhi high court's judgment, which decriminalizes homosexual relationships, has created a sort of uproar among religious leaders. Religious leaders like Reverend Dominic Emmanuel, spokesperson of the Delhi Catholic Archdiocese said: "the Catholic Church has nothing against gays, but we strongly believe that sex between same sex partners is immoral, unnatural and unethical".

His counterpart in Mumbai, Rev. Tony Charanghat, observed: "While homosexuals have to be treated with respect, homosexuality can't be equated with heterosexuality. The nature of sex should be complementary to life, which is God's design".

In fact, Mumbai's catholic secular forum (CSF) circulated mass SMS appealing to Catholics to protest against the move to legalize homosexuality. "We protest on both health and religious grounds", says Joseph Dias, CSF General Secretary. "We have statistics to prove that a large number of HIV cases are gay, and this verdict may lead to an AIDS epidemic of sort," Dias added.

Yoga teacher Swami Ramdev minced no words. "Do the people behind this verdict consider homosexuality natural? Is it something they will themselves do? If our parents had been gays, could we have born? Freedom doesn't mean license. Our family system is the ideal system which we can show to the world. Sadly, this judgment will end up corrupting it. I will be a part of protest against the judgment: Baba Ramdev further commented: "These (gays) are sick people and should be sent to hospitals. Then they can marry or stay as bachelors just like me" - This statement expresses total disrespect to gay community by Ram Dev Baba.

Muslim clerics in both Mumbai and Delhi expressed shock. India is a secular state, but most of the Indians are religious minded people, and no religion allows homosexuality. If homosexuality is legalized, it will damage our culture and value system. 'There should be a parliamentary debate and more stringent laws to discourage people and to avoid unnatural sex," said Maulana Mehmood Madani, general secretary, Jamiat lemma-e Hind.

Guyana Graham Singh, a Sikh leader and head priest of Akal Tact, reacted sharply and said: 'We oppose this decision. It's against the law of nature. We appeal to the Government to rethink on the issue. We also ask the Sikh community to boycott this verdict, as it is against to the teachings of Guru Granth Sahib."[7]

By and large all religious groups have made it clear that they consider gay sex "immoral and anti-religion", and they expect the government to appeal the order. Most of the chief religious heads in the country opposed any legalization in favour of homosexuality as it negates their belief, but that belief can not prevent sex between two gays and hidden dangers of HIV transmission and sexually transmitted diseases. Therefore, the government stand should be supported in the interest of the health of the homosexuals.

Government Not to Appeal Against Court Judgment:

Health minister Ghulam Nabi Azad took a strictly non-committal approach, indicating apprehensions over the conservative reaction. With gay rights becoming a hot debate, the Government is relieved from the pressures of the religious leaders and it need not go for any legislation against homosexuality. The government may maintain neutrality between the anger of religious leaders and the progressive opinion of the public.

Azad has already said there is need for a debate in parliament and in other forums before the government could consider its position on gay sex. Indicating the pulls and pressures exerted by vocal groups on both sides, Ms. Giraja Vyas, chairperson of the National commission for women, echoed the view that the issue is needed "widest consultation." Referring to homosexuality she said: 'We believe if sex is forced, it is rape. But consensual sex between two adults of the same gender may be seen as unnatural by same sections, we must consider that too".

Apart from the social aspects of the law, the government is also considering the arguments that legalizing homosexuality might make it easier to tackle HIV in a highly vulnerable section that has been driven undergrounds.[8]

Spread of HIV/AIDS:

The hidden nature of homosexual groups is impeding intervention under the National AIDS Control Programme. A suitable environment is to be created where the people who involve in risky behavior could have total access to the use of services for such behaviour to prevent themselves from risky factors.

The court verdict also has implications for heterosexuals, as all consensual sexual acts of adults in private are legalized. Earlier, oral and anal sexes were treated as unnatural and punishable under the same section. Rejecting the argument of the council for Home Ministry that homosexuality was mental disease, the judges said that it was "just another expression of human sexuality."

The court accepted the petitioner's (a Non-Government Organisation) NGO argument that criminalization of homosexual acts severely hampered the AIDS intervention programs. The NGO had argued that the fear of harassment by law enforcement authority leads to hurried sex, leaving the partners without the option to consider or negotiate the safer sex practices. It also said that the hidden nature of gay groups further led to poor access to condom, health care services, and safe sex information.

Nazi Foundation's argument was reinforced by 2006 statistics submitted by National AIDS Control Organization that 8 per cent of the 25 lakh homosexuals in India were infected with HIV, while its prevalence among general population was less than one per cent. "An enabling environment needs to be created where people involved in risky behavior are encouraged not to conceal information so that they can be provided total access to the services of such preventive efforts said the high court".[9]

Misconceptions that Handicap Society:

Legalizing the Lesbian Gay Bisexual Transgender (LGBT) relationships has two entirely divergent angles. It is both an issue of religious faith as well as a matter of human rights. Unfortunately, as a bystander, I have seen more than one occasion that religious beliefs and human rights do not go hand in hand. Our experiences with the Talibans in Afghanistan and the Catholic Church's view against abortion and several other instances have more than ample evidence to prove the point.

In such a situation, how can we expect major religions of this country would go all out to embrace the LGBT community with open arms? Not at all. Hinduism disagrees with those who indulge in homosexual relationships. Islam prohibits homosexual relationships.

Islam also prohibits alcohol, eating pork and idol worship. Should Muslims go to the government to ban all these activities?

Matter of Human Rights:

In legalizing gay rights in India, the Delhi High Court has shown its utter acceptance of a community, which has long been shunning in our society. The court order is accommodating those who live a life as they think is good and natural for them. If we cannot accept this change, then we should have reservations on orders prohibiting "sati" (self-burning of widows) and "child marriage". Supporting the legalization of gay rights does not mean to encouraging this practice, but accepting the rights of persons who constitute a section of our society.

It is wrongly felt that the Delhi High Court has opened the flood gates for such relationships. On hearing the court order "Oh my God, my son will be a gay now", shouted a man in an interview on a TV channel. I wish I could tell him that his son will be a gay or a heterosexual not because of the high Court order but because of his sons' sexual orientation and preferences.

These are misconceptions that handicap society from accepting a change. Good or bad, change is the law of nature and social changes need to manifest their full impact.[10] By and large, a hidden practice of homosexuality in the country is legalized so that their health will be protected.

Truck Drivers' Lifestyle and HIV/AIDS:

The truck drivers or the long distance lorry drivers are a specialized group because of their work culture. India has one of the largest road networks in the world and an estimated five million long distance truck driver in the country. These men are away from their families for long durations due to lengthy journey from days to weeks and months. Day and night driving along the highways in a detrimental environment, the truck drivers become easy prey for commercial sex workers. Hence, this background has brought new dimensions to their lifestyle. A recent study of Thai long distance truck drivers found that 86% of the single men and 63% of the married men had had commercial sex[11]. Some activists vehemently opposed to use the word commercial sex worker or commercial sex, and the promiscuous behaviour of truck drivers and so on. Obviously we can not label this group is bad and that group is good etc.,

During their journeys, long distance truck drivers stop at "dhabas," (road side hotels), which usually provide food, rest, sex workers, alcohol, and drugs. They pick up the women, use them and leave them at some other dhaba. The dabhas are the road side hotels and motels, which are used by other drivers and local youths. Thus long distance lorry drivers are crucial in spreading sexually transmitted diseases and HIV infection throughout the country in short time. They have an HIV infection rate of 10/1000, far higher than the Indian national average of bout 0.5/1000.[12] In our study we found that the drivers aged above 40 years were highly vulnerable, and potential for transmission of sexually transmitted diseases .This group is the most threatening. Though their knowledge of AIDS is fairly good, their use of condoms is poor and it is 11% only. As in Tanzania[13], condom use should be promoted along truck routs by distributing condoms freely through condom outlets[14]. In other studies the incidence of HIV was 23% among Indian truck drivers and 56% in African truck drivers visiting sex workers in KwaZulu-Natal, South Africa[15]. In another research in Andhra Pradesh, India at baseline, 2.1% of drivers were HIV infected and 34% reported having contact with female sex workers (FSWs) within the previous six months[16]. For that reason research is urgently needed to find effective strategies to persuade truck drivers to change their hazardous sexual behavior to prevent HIV among them.

"HIV is not a burden; poverty is", as told by Phool Chand, a 36 year old truck driver. To his mind poverty is a more burden than HIV and perhaps he thinks that he can conquer HIV if he has enough money. He worked in West Bengal for more than six years and he moved to Jalpaiguri where he worked as a driver of local passengers' bus and subsequently joined in a school to drive their van which he feels it as a less stressful job. He became positive while he was working on Mumbai-Goa highway. In an interview he said: "What had to happen has happened. Now the only thing that matters for me is to take my medicines on time. It is important that the treatment for HIV be free of cost. Also it would be thoughtful on the government's part to provide us with a life insurance policy that can benefit our family once we are no more. Free schooling to children and a minimum pension to the surviving spouse would be a relief too. I wonder the life insurance for HIV/AIDS patients in this country is still a daydream".

He continued that "some sort of assurance would be necessary, that the school employer's should not discontinue my services in case they know my HIV positive state. As my condition worsens, I am likely to need few days leave from time to time. Most employers are not very tolerant." He also told: "majority of the times a truck driver is on a long drive; fatigue, loneliness and the fear of death are his constant companions. It gets extremely monotonous and boring. It is very painful to be away from our wives and families for long stretches of time."[17]

To overcome such painful experiences of truck drivers, I have made a suggestion, to the government of India to start rest homes for truck drivers on highways so that they can have recreation, food, health care tips and safety measures, and safe sex guidelines through these homes. But unfortunately so far no such positive steps have been initiated by the government in this direction.

AIDS – Ethical Issues:

Since the HIV epidemic continues to exert a heavy toll in India and world over, numerous health related legal, ethical, and human rights problems are being encountered in the process. Therefore, in the wake of the discrimination suffered by individuals with HIV/AIDS and their partners and families, now more attention has been focused on them.

During the early years of the epidemic, the most common legislative approach required is the notification of persons with AIDS to the public health authorities.[18] While case reporting has contributed to the efforts to monitor the evolving epidemic; the reporting systems in some countries are not structured around the concept of confidentiality. As a result, the identity of infected persons becomes a matter of the public domain. With growing pressures to protect the identity of infected persons, some countries have updated their notification laws, but quite a large number of countries still continuing the same practice.[19] In India the VCTC (Voluntary Counseling and testing centers) strictly maintain the confidentiality of positive people. All social problems are moral problems. Due to social stigma attached to AIDS, doctors usually change the names of the patients to avoid identity of the person in the society.

In addition to several legal problems, the HIV/AIDS epidemic has been posing a variety of ethical challenges in matters concerning maintaining confidentiality, to get informed consent of the patient before testing and initiating treatment; counseling of women to make reproductive decisions, burden on the infected individuals to protect their sexual partners, issues related to research and care, the social stigma attached to it, obligations of the state to prevent spread of the disease, obligations on the part of physicians to care for HIV infected with due respect to them, issues related to insurance, responsibility of developed countries to assist the developing countries, and rights of HIV infected men, women and children. The threat of AIDS has provided a platform to rethink about our traditional approach to public health in the light of human rights, and the dignity and worthiness of human life.

Moral Responsibility of HIV Infected:

In India, about 86% of HIV transmissions are through heterosexual route. And the rest are through contaminated needles, sharing of needle and syringes by IV drug users, pregnant mother to the infant and accidental exposure of health care providers while providing care to HIV infected patients. Homosexual route is also contributing silently to the spread of HIV. The accidental exposure while providing care to HIV infected is the biggest issue in the medical circles now. While treating HIV/AIDS patients and admitting them in the hospitals, several administrative difficulties and sensitive matters are coming up. In the earlier periods when the AIDS epidemic was identified, the nurses refused to attend on them and they went on mass strike in Kerala, Madurai and other parts of the country. Not to admit an HIV patient in the hospital and treat him properly, is a violation of his rights. The government instructions are clearly in favour of admitting HIV positive people in general wards along with the other patients and to treat them like any other patient. The question involved here is, whether the medical and paramedical staff and the menial staff are given the required training to deal safely with HIV positive patients. If it is not so, what would be the consequences?

The world Health organization and the government of India are advocating universal precautions to be followed at work place. Is there enough funding for creating awareness and supervision to prevent spread of HIV? It is an open secret that many hospitals are refusing to admit HIV positive patients. At this point, there is a conflict between Hypocritic Oath and the attitude of health care providers and hospitals. For example, when I was studying in Christian Medical College, Vellore, I have come across a young post graduate student sustained needle stick injury while giving intravenous (IV) injection to a known HIV positive patient. Imagine the psychological stress and tension of that student, though drugs were available at that time free of cost for post exposure prophylaxis at Christian Medical College, Vellore. But how many Government Hospitals are providing the regular supply of ART for post exposure prophylaxis (PEP) is a matter of concern to the health care providers.

One day it was so happened that a staff nurse broke into tears when she had gush of blood on her face while she was engaged in conducting the delivery on HIV positive woman. In such circumstances, the health care providers discharge their duties to the AIDS patients at a greater risk of being infected and thus HIV becomes a professional hazard.[20]

Ethical Issues in the Use of Condoms:

Extensive studies in Thailand have proved beyond doubt that proper use of condoms significantly reduces the risk of transmission of HIV. Thailand is a country, whose major source of income is from tourism, especially from call girls and hence the whole country accustomed to implement vigorously the use of condoms. Even the

Health Minister of Thailand used to carry condoms and distributed to the people who are in need of them. Campaign of this high magnitude attracted the attention of the globe and many countries started campaigning condoms to prevent AIDS. WHO and UNAIDS also recommended the use of condoms to prevent AIDS. Use of condoms on a large scale raises some ethical issues. The religious leaders of all major religions of the world opposed use of condoms for the reason that they provoke and encourage illegal and immoral contacts and spoil the youth.

Reaction to Pope's Remarks:

AIDS Healthcare Foundation (AHF) admonished the Pope for his claim that condoms were not a solution to the AIDS epidemic. In his remarks to a group of reporters en route to Africa, Pope Benedict said: "AIDS is a tragedy that cannot be overcome by money alone, and that cannot be overcome through the distribution of condoms, rather it aggravates the problem."

Dr. George Saavedra, Chief of Global Affairs for AIDS Healthcare Foundation said: "Governments are obligated to follow scientific evidence in order to set up effective public health policies to fight AIDS and not rely on religious beliefs like the one Pope Benedict is promoting." He also remarks: "One day, or may be one hundred years from now, the Catholic Church is going to apologize for these kinds of statements, the same way they did several hundred years after the inquisition and half a century after the Holocaust."

Terri Ford, Senior Director of Global Policy for AHF said: "Some governments, as well as families, if they follow the Pope's directive, then literally people will die, leaving more orphans. Surely that is not God's plan." He also stated: "As the leader of the Catholic Church, Pope Benedict certainly has the right to express his opposition to the use of condoms on moral grounds, but when he deliberately distorts the widely-recognized and respected scientific findings about the efficacy of condoms in slowing the spread of the AIDS virus, he creates unnecessary impediments in the global fight against the epidemic, which becomes a great threat to human lives. The Pope must be reminded that those kinds of statements cost lives."

Whitney Engeran-Cordova, Director of AIDS Healthcare Foundation's Public Health Division said: "The Pope should be offering constructive real world solutions to the global AIDS epidemic and not distracting us from the single most effective prevention tool we have today, condoms." Condoms can cost as little as three cents a piece. If the Vatican truly wants to contribute in the global fight against AIDS, it should offer more constructive input and solutions. For those of us in the fight against AIDS every day, we simply cannot rely on such old world thinking in managing this 21st century epidemic."[21]

Pope's Approach to Control AIDS:

Pope Benedict XVI in his week-long trip to the continent said: "Condoms are not the answer to Africa's fight against HIV". It was the pope's first explicit statement on an issue that has divided even clergy working with AIDS patients. Benedict arrived in Yaoundé, Cameroon's capital, where he was, greeted by a crowd of flag-waving faithful and snapping cameras. In his four years as Pope, Benedict had never directly addressed condom use, although his position is not new. His predecessor, Pope John Paul II, often said that sexual abstinence -- not condoms -- was the best way to prevent the spread of the disease.

Benedict also said that the Roman Catholic Church was at the forefront of the battle against AIDS. "You can't resolve it with the distribution of condoms. On the contrary, it increases the problem." The pope said that a responsible and moral attitude towards sex would help to fight the disease. The Roman Catholic Church rejects the use of condoms as part of its overall teaching against artificial contraception. Senior Vatican officials have advocated fidelity in marriage and abstinence from premarital sex as key weapons in the fight against AIDS.

According to UNAIDS about 22 million people in sub-Saharan Africa are infected with HIV. Rebecca Hodes, with the Treatment Action Campaign in South Africa, said: "If the Pope was serious about preventing new HIV infections, he would focus on promoting wide access to condoms and spreading information on how best to use them. Instead, his opposition to condoms conveys that religious dogma is more important to him than the lives of Africans." Even some priests and nuns working with those living with HIV/AIDS question the church's opposition to condoms amid the pandemic ravaging Africa. Many Africans were of the opinion, "Talking about the non-use of condoms is out of place. We need condoms to protect ourselves against HIV and AIDS," said a teacher Ms. Narcisse Takou in Yaoundé.[22]

The Reaction of IAS on Pope's Remarks on Condoms:

Julio Montaner, President of the International AIDS Society (IAS) has described that the comments made by Pope Benedict XVI's on the role of condoms as "irresponsible and dangerous". He said: "There is not a shred of evidence to suggest that condoms can increase HIV transmission and the Pope's statement is absolutely the contrary." Male and female condoms, used correctly and consistently, can reduce the risk of sexual transmission of HIV by 80-90 percent.

IAS Executive Director Craig McClure further condemned the Pope's remarks. "To suggest that condom use contributes to the HIV problem is not merely contrary to scientific evidence and global consensus, but it contributes to fueling HIV infection and its consequences are sickness and death. Such outrageous comments are not appropriate coming from the highest office in the hierarchy of the Catholic Church." Dr. Montaner added that while condoms are not the only solution to combating HIV, they are a critical, cheap, and cost-effective element of a comprehensive approach to HIV prevention. Instead of spreading ignorance, the Pope should use his global position of leadership to encourage young people, who are our future, to protect themselves and others from HIV infection using all the tools we have at our disposal, including condoms.

His remarks are insulting to the tireless efforts of committed scientific, public health and human rights leaders around the world to protect the poorest of the poor from HIV infection.

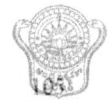

The IAS is the world leading association of HIV professionals, with more than 13,000 members from 188 countries working at all levels of the global response to HIV/AIDS. IAS members represent scientists, clinicians, and public health and community practitioners on the front lines of the epidemic.[9] As a member of IAS for the last several years, I had an opportunity to contribute the best available input from this region for its leadership.

Condoms and HIV Prevention Efforts:

Condoms are an integral and essential part of HIV prevention and care programmes, and their promotion must be accelerated says, the Global Network of People Living with HIV/AIDS (GNP+) and the International Network of Religious Leaders Living with or personally affected by HIV/AIDS. Abstinence and mutual fidelity are highly effective means of reducing sexual exposure to HIV, but they must be promoted within a comprehensive prevention strategy that includes all effective methods. Condoms are an essential part of this overall strategy."

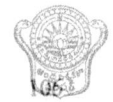

Kevin Moody, International Coordinator and CEO of GNP+ concurred: "Condoms are an essential tool in promoting, attaining and maintaining the sexual and reproductive health of everyone, including people living with HIV. Over a quarter of a century into the epidemic, it is sad that we are still debating whether or not condoms should be part of the prevention effort." Conclusive evidence from extensive research among heterosexual couples in which one partner is HIV positive shows that correct and consistent condom use significantly reduces the risk of HIV transmission from men to women, and also from women to men.

In the research conducted by GNP+ with serodiscordant couples in South Africa, Tanzania and Ukraine the majority of couples indicated consistent condom use as their strategy for practicing safer sex. As the search for new HIV prevention technologies such as Microbicides and vaccines continues to progress, scaling-up access to male and female condoms is essential in addressing HIV prevention needs of all people. In addition to increasing the availability and accessibility of condoms, HIV prevention requires a comprehensive approach which includes access to accurate information, access to HIV treatment, harm reduction measures, confronting stigma and discrimination, affirming faith communities and ensuring a supportive legal and political environment for people living with HIV.[23]

Use of Microbicides to Prevent HIV:

A Microbicide is any substance that can substantially reduce the transmission of sexually transmitted infections (STIs) when applied either in the vagina or rectum. A Microbicide could be produced in many forms, including gels, creams, suppositories, films, lubricants or in the form of a sponge or a vaginal ring that slowly releases the active ingredient over time. The word "Microbicides" refers to a range of different products that share one common characteristic, the ability to prevent the sexual transmission of HIV and other STI pathogens when applied topically. Researchers at the London School of Hygiene and Tropical Medicine have used epidemiological models to estimate the number of HIV infections that could be averted as a result of Microbicide use, and the numbers are impressive. Basing on conservative assumptions, the model examined the impact of introducing a Microbicide in 73 under developed and developing countries. The model assumes that the product is used by 20% of individuals who can be reached through existing services, and that it is used in 50% of sex acts where condoms are not used.[24]

A Catholic Bishop of South Africa Accepts the Use of Condoms:

It is good that one of the Catholic bishops of South Africa says 'yes' to the use of condoms. Kevin Dowling is the Catholic Bishop of Rustenburg, South Africa, a mining town where 50% of pregnant women test positive for HIV. In 1998, he started "Tapologo", a community-centered HIV/AIDS programme, which provides home-based care, antiretroviral therapy, and in-patient care at a hospice. "We are trying to empower the women to have some say over their sexual lives, but that's not easy when they're dependent on sex for survival. There's no way that women are going to be saved from certain death in this area unless they're economically and educationally empowered. The socio-economic and cultural realities would bring major success with behaviour modification. It is very small, even though we continue to try." He further told: "I think the issue, then, comes down to: 'what is the best available means we have to protect life?' and at the moment it is only the condom. It's in conflict with the official Catholic Church position, but I've reflected on this for many years and I truly feel that in the case of this hyper-epidemic, the issue is, in the end, very simple: preservation and protection of life. The best available means we have to protect life is the condom."

"The Pope is, after all, not a public health expert and his views on condoms should not be given space. He is, however, right about responsibility, though he would not agree with these words: a much greater number of people need to practice safer sex if we are to defeat HIV. That includes the use of condoms with every partner. But safer sex is also a way of thinking and acting towards one's partner(s). It is about openness, communication, respect and mutual protection as well as shared pleasure. Right now, HIV is still winning. For me, the bigger issue is: why are most of us still not putting more effort into promoting prevention and condoms,"? Commented Ms. Marge Berer on Pope's statement.[25]

A top medical research journal Lancet urged Pope Benedict XVI to take back his "distorting" comments on the use of condoms in the fight against HIV/AIDS disease during his recent Africa tour where he said that HIV / AIDS was "a tragedy that cannot be overcome by money alone, which cannot be overcome through the distribution of condoms, which can even increase the problem". Pope further suggested that the "cruel epidemic" should be tackled through abstinence and fidelity rather than condom use.

The Lancet, regarded as one of the world's most prestigious medical journals, said the remarks were "wildly inaccurate" and could have "devastating consequences." In its unprecedented attack, described as "virulent" by commentators, the Lancet said the Pope had "publicly distorted scientific evidence to promote Catholic doctrine on this issue". "Whether the Pope's error was due to ignorance or a deliberate attempt to manipulate science to support Catholic ideology is unclear," said the journal.

"When any influential person, be it a religious or political figure, makes a false scientific statement that could be devastating to the health of millions of people, they should retract or correct the public record," it said.

"Anything less from Pope Benedict would be an immense disservice to the public and health advocates, including many thousands of Catholics, who work tirelessly to try and prevent the spread of HIV/AIDS worldwide.

The Pope's remarks were condemned by the governments of Germany, France and Belgium and by aid organizations. UNAIDS, the UN Population Fund, and the World Health Organization (WHO) released statements defending the use of condoms as the "single, most efficient, available tool.[26] The religious beliefs of Pope and his comments on condom were almost challenged by scientists, research workers and academicians.

Under this background some orthodox people raised moral questioner such as should we encourage multiple sexual partners or prostitution by promoting condom use? Is it not unethical to have extramarital sex or prostitution by using condoms?

There is a strong criticism against the use of condoms on the ground that it is shaking the sacredness of marriage bond between a man and a woman. In the name of AIDS, multinational companies like Hindustan Latex is manufacturing and supplying millions of condoms and it is spoiling the youth of this country.

Monogamy is the fundamental fabric of Indian culture and it is at greater risk due to free supply of condoms. Thus, the latex rubber sheath has shaken the sacred sheath of Indian couples and the marriage bond between them. Sex for pleasure is a bygone saying in the AIDS ruled world. Even if we image sexual act for the sake of pleasure, it is creating scare in the minds of people. There is a belief that God created AIDS to check the unethical behaviour of promiscuity and to control the mushroom growth of population.

Kama or desire for pleasure is one of the cardinal values of Hindu ethics. Sex is considered as one of the basic human instincts that agitate human being. Hindu ethical thinkers recognized the rightful satisfaction of sexual desire within proper limits, which ensures bodily and mental health of the individual.

Hindu thinkers never preached the negation of sex. But sexual desire deprived of righteousness is a mere lust, and it gives rise to various kinds of vices. It not only degrades one's character, but also disturbs the social and moral order of the society. A person highly indulgent in sexual desire loses his rational thinking and fails to understand what is good and what is bad. If one becomes a slave of sexual pleasure, he brings his own destruction. Mahabharata recognizes four vices which make a man lose his rationality. They are hunting, addiction to drink, love of gambling and too much love for the company of women.[27]

The problem of HIV/AIDS is closely linked to a person's excessive desire for sexual pleasure. If a man or a woman is in the lust for excessive sexual pleasure, they may be vulnerable to HIV virus infection.

Unethical Vengeance:

It has come to knowledge that some of the positive patients with a vengeance on the society in a psychological depressive mood are infecting the innocent negative women by hiding their positive status. Is it not unethical to infect a woman by a man or vice-versa? This sort of behaviour is a big crime and a 'time bomb' to the community.

Depressed mood and loss of interest and pleasure characterize these disorders. If they alternate with exaggerated elation or irritability they are known as by polar disorders (one pole, depressed; another pole, elation or mania). The severity symptoms that often accompany the depressed mood, and the duration of the disorder differentiates them from normal mood changes.

The causes of these disorders vary, and there may be psycho-social risk factors that influence the onset and persistence of the depressive episodes or biological factors of different kinds. Studies demonstrate that one out of seven adult persons of the USA has a mood disorder during a single year, 7% in Brazil, almost 10% in Germany and 4.2% in Turkey. Ignoring this reality can result in suicide. Depressive disorders and schizophrenia are responsible for

60% of all suicides.[28] HIV virus itself cause depression and mood disorders so positive persons at times behave so erratically and may infect intentionally many innocent persons.

Ethics and Prevention of AIDS:

HIV is basically a behaviorally transmitted disease, and transmission of HIV can be prevented or interrupted through a proper modification of human behaviour viz., using condom during sexual intercourse, not sharing needles by IV drug users, and using therapeutic intervention by pregnant women to reduce mother to child transmission of HIV etc.,

Though it's the moral responsibility of the HIV infected persons to develop a responsible behaviour to control the spread, but in practice it is utterly lacking. The government while designing preventive policies should be conscious of facilitating the modification of sexual and drug abuse behaviour. The factors need to be debated to prevent sexual transmission of HIV includes the empowerment of women to make safer sexual relationships in the light of their culture and heritage. The AIDS prevention efforts that are not culturally sensitive and that ignore the local issues, will fail to reach the intended people. In fact, they may create opposite force to the implementation of the programme.

The fundamental principles of ethics demand that individuals, even if they are HIV positives should be treated with respect and their dignity as human beings should be protected. Since AIDS carries a discomfort stigma, many positives are being isolated from society, deprived of active public life, and some of them are going underground, and a few sensitive individuals are even committing suicides. This will depict the magnitude of the problem. Therefore, there is a tremendous responsibility on the part of medical and paramedical personnel to maintain secrecy about the persons affected by AIDS.

On the "World AIDS Day", that is, December 1, 1999, The Times magazine in its cover story published the headlines as "LOSING BATTLE AGAINST AIDS." A young positive of 22 years old, after seeing the caption, committed suicide with a suicide note to his brother states: "I expected a cure for AIDS, but none other than the Times magazine published an article on "losing battle against AIDS", and it clearly indicates that I got a disease which has no cure." The slain brother wrote a letter to the editor of Times magazine stating that "Your caption on AIDS killed my brother. Please don't play with sensitive guys". Hence it is said that "media created more scare than care" about AIDS. Unless the journalists and publishing houses maintain a code of conduct, and follow media ethics while reporting stories on burning issues like AIDS, an unrepairable damage will be done to the society. In the process of creating awareness on HIV / AIDS, overenthusiastic journalism becomes a massacre of sensitive, emotional and innocent people. It needs a critical retrospection and suitable corrective measures immediately in publishing news on sensitive issues.

Summary:

The legal and moral issues involved in HIV/AIDS at every level viz., from the point of diagnosis to till death and also after death are highly sensitive, sentimental and complex. In view of this the government is interfering from time to time to safeguard the rights of PLWAs. And AIDS activists are also protesting whenever justice is denied to them. In spite of this HIV infected are facing humiliation and termination of their employment once their employer identifies them. This attitude becomes a big blow on several young, energetic, positive persons as they fail to get a right job and fail to continue in the job respectfully. The fundamental principles of ethics demand that HIV positive persons should be treated with respect and dignity as human beings.

In other situations where positive people are working knowingly to the customers in public outlets like canteens or bakery, the management fears that they may loose their business. Even hospitals are afraid to admit positive people as their presence may not allow normal patients to come to that hospital for treatment. In practice, it is true that some hospitals suffered severe losses and drastic fall in admissions of general patients. There are also reports that due to lack of customers some hotels and departmental stores were closed because the customers come to know that HIV positive persons are working as stewards and sales girls in those establishments.

In recent times, sexuality and sexual rights of gay community have come into frontline, as section 377 of the IPC, which criminalize consensual sexual acts of adults in private, was struck down by the Delhi High Court. Though this act brought mixed reactions from the various groups of people, it will certainly prevent HIV among homosexuals as they will come out to the main stream of public life without fear or diffidence and participate in the AIDS prevention programs.

As condoms remain critical in HIV prevention, several international AIDS working groups such as IAS and (AHF) AIDS health care foundation opposed on the comments of Pope Benedict, who stated that AIDS can not be overcome through the distribution of condoms, rather it aggravates the problem. But the scientific outcome based on several research studies indicates that condom is one of the best available means we have to protect life.

It was narrated in the Bhagavad-Gita by the Lord Krishna that if people can control their sexual desires and lust, the chastity will be maintained. Then the question of condom use may not arise. But how far it is practicable? As long as the extramarital sex, multiple sex partners, exchange of partners, prostitution and sexual exploitation shall continue, so long HIV will flourish. Therefore, there is an urgent need for modification in human sexual behaviour.

References:

1. The Hindu, Legal Correspondent, October 2, 2008.
2. The Hindu, Legal Correspondent, Sunday, July 29, 2008.
3. A living history of AIDS vaccine research 'IAVI report', March – April 2009, Vol. 13, No.2, P 8-9.
4. Targeted Genetics Corporation [homepage on the internet]. Targeted Genetics announces preliminary safety data from phase-I HIV vaccine trial. [Cited 2007 Jan 8]. Available from:

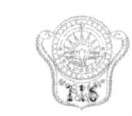

"*http://ir.targen.com/* phoenix.zhtml? C" c=84981 & p=irol_news Articles & ID=677299 & highlight.

5. Manoj mitta & Smriti Singh-Times of India FRIDAY, JULY 3, 2009-P. 1

6. Kounteya Sinha, Times of India New Delhi FRIDAY, JULY 3, 2009-P. 9

7. The times of India New Delhi, July 3 2009 P. 12

8. The Times of India New Delhi FRIDAY, JULY 3, 2009-P. 10

9. Harish V Nair: Hindustan times-Friday, July 3, 2009-P. 1

10. The Hindu: Sunday, July 19, 2009-P. 19

11. Bloom DE, Lyons JV, "Behavior pattern of Thai long haul truck drivers": Institute for population and social Research, Mahidol University, Bangkok, *"Economic implications of AIDS in Asia"*. New Delhi; UNDP Regional Bureau for Asia and the pacific, 1993:80-1.

12. Singh YN, Singh K, Joshi R, Rustagi GK, Malaviya AN. HIV infection among long distance truck drivers in Delhi India; *"AIDS and Asia: a development crisis"*. New Delhi Department of Medicine, All India Institute of Medical Science, 1992. (UNDP) Regional Project on HIV/AIDS.

13. Huddart j. *"HIV in the work place: Dealing with issues-role plays"*. Boston: United Nations Development Programme, 1993.

14. Kutikuppala Surya Rao, et. al.: Sexual lifestyle of long distance lorry drivers in India: *"British Medical Journal (BMJ)"* Vol.:318 16 January 999 P162-163

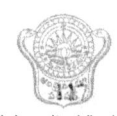

15. Ramjee.G and Gouws.E ,Medical Research Council, , *"HIV prevention among truck drivers"* South Africa: Global Development Network" *2010 P-1*

16. 20.J.A.Schneider , A. Dude et al., *"International Journal of STD & AIDS"* (The Royal Society of Medicine Press, London UK Volume 20, Number 1, 2009) pp. 39-45

17. Positive Space, *"NACO NEWS"*, A newsletter of the National AIDS Control Organization, Vol. 5, Issue 2, April-June 2009, P. 14-15.

18. Fluss S.S. *"National AIDS Legislation: An overview of Some Global Developments"* in Gostin, L. and L. Porter (eds.) International Law and AIDS: International Responses, Current Issues, and Future Directions, American Bar Association, Chicago, 1992, p. 15-17.

19. DC Jayasuriya, *"HIV Law: The Expanding Frontiers*, HIV Law Ethics and Human Rights Chapter 1: pp. 9-10.

20. Usha K. Bavaja *"Legal and ethical issues of HIV/AIDS"* "Diagnosis and Management of HIV/AIDS, A Clinician's Perspective", B.I Publications Pvt Ltd, New Delhi 2005, p.405.

21. Victor L. Simpson http:// ga1.org/ join-forward. html? Domain =Aids health&r=a1xMNUn 1rkSH, *"Pope Says Condoms Worsen HIV Problem"* : Associated Press, March 18, 2009.

22. http://www.washingtonpost.com/wpdyn/content/article/ 2009 /03 /17/AR2009031703369.html

23. Karen Bennett (Geneva, Switzerland) IAS Senior Communications Manager Info & archives: http:// list. Healt hnet.org / mailman / listinfo / procaare.

24. Martin Stolk, Communications Officer: GNP+ International Secretariat Email: mstolk@gnpplus.net. www.inerela.org, press release-20 March 2009.

25. Kutikuppala Surya Rao, World AIDS Day-2004, "The Antiseptic" Estd. 1904, Vol. 101 No. 12, December 2004, p. 556.

26. Marge Berer Editor, *"Reproductive Health Matters"*. Web: www.rhmjournal.org.uk-IRINPlus News, 22 August 2008.

27. Kamala Subrahmaniam, *"Mahabharata"*, (Bombay, Bharatiya Vidhya Bhavan, 1995) p. 169.

28. Kutikuppala Surya Rao, Special article: Mental Health around the World, *"JIMA, Journal of the Indian Medical Association"*, Volume 99, Number 4, April 2001, p. 218.

Chapter Five

AIDS Care Physicians and Society Perception

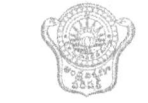

CHAPTER - V

AIDS CARE PHYSICIANS AND SOCIETY PERCEPTION

In the early years of AIDS epidemic the hospital staff used to leave food trays and plates at the doors of patients who are sick of AIDS. The nurses, physicians and dentists also refused to attend on patients suffering from this new disease. In those days, it was so happened because the mode of transmission of the disease was not clear, and thus people were very much scared of AIDS. During this time the (CDC) centers for disease control confronted with such behaviours. But in the late 1985 and 1986, a series of reports were published in the morbidity and mortality weekly report (MMWR), which provided guidance for sound infection control practice and rational societal policy. Thus the lack of knowledge about spreading of AIDS frightened physicians and health care workers, and they used to consider their profession as a dangerous trade.[1]

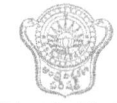

Though the health care workers in the USA and other advanced industrial countries had experience of treating the sick for about four decades with the acquisition of their patients' infections and sometimes lethal diseases, it has never been as total as many had to come to believe this invincibility was psychologically ruptured by the intrusion of AIDS reported in 1981. However, some of the physicians who were committed to face the situation had a hope that clear guidelines would emerge in due course to deal with AIDS patients.[2]

Physicians happened to be the frontline force and they used to respond whenever some epidemics outburst, which cause deadly sickness among people. The experiences of the past showed that many health care providers are scarred and escaped to attend epidemics, though some physicians had stayed behind to care for the patients. After all a physician is also a human being, and thus he/she has their inherited attitudes, fears, apprehensions, sentiments, superstitions, pains, pleasures, and so on. Medical profession is something which is opted by them. Unless a person is highly committed to the profession and decided to sacrifice his/her life for the cause of suffering, coming forward to treat infected patients like HIV/AIDS, he or she is not a true doctor. At times, doctors may hesitate to treat HIV positive patients simply to protect themselves from the infection. This is almost a reflection of the plague era, where separate arrangements were made to take care of the plague patients through special institutions. 'Plague Doctors' were employed specially by the local merchants and the political elite when other physicians refused to treat plague cases. The situation of AIDS now is worse than the days of plague.

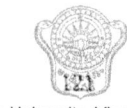

Hence, policy makers and public health experts are struggling with this issue to guarantee each HIV infected individual to have sound access to health care. Ethics of care encompasses providing medical services to the HIV infected without discrimination and at the same time maintaining the confidentiality.[3] Several arguments came about the care of the AIDS patients such as "individual responsibility" of health care worker, and collective responsibility of medical profession. However, the aim is that a holistic approach and a team work should be implemented while treating a complex disease like AIDS.[4] In short, some people argue that as long as the needs of the HIV infected are completely met, there is no valid reason for insisting that each health care worker should share the responsibility.

Is it morally right to the medical staff to refuse to attend on HIV/AIDS patients? Due to the seriousness of AIDS disease, even today many physicians, surgeons, gynecologists, obstetricians, nursing staff, and paramedical personnel are reluctant to attend on HIV positive patients. Historically, a sudden appearance of any new fatal epidemic creates some fear, and the transmissible nature of this fatal disease has escalated fear to phobia as public dread of AIDS spreads rapidly not only throughout America, but all over the world.[5]

Public fear is largely a curious mixture of homo phobia and the fear of catching AIDS through casual contact. This is because of unprecedented awareness created on the rumors and false stories of HIV/AIDS, rather than the scientific facts about AIDS. The following events illustrate the real picture of AIDS

Andhra University, Visakhapatnam

For instance, an AIDS patient arrived at North Carolina Memorial Hospital from another small hospital, in a body bag normally used to ship a corpse. The duty Nurse, Suzi reported the matter to the doctors. At the top of the bag there was a small air tube so that the patient could breathe. When the nurse unzipped the bag, the patient blinked. "He was alert and well oriented".[6] However, the way in which the AIDS patient was brought to the hospital was miserable and inhuman.

In the second case the Delta Airlines proposed a rule to forbid carrying AIDS patients. (The proposal was dropped in February 1985).[7] However, the proposal itself is a serious blow on the rights of HIV positive people.

In a third issue, a telephone company attempted to sell disposable telephones for AIDS patients to hospitals in Arkansas (USA). A sales brochure recommended that "Patients be told when they are admitted that they must purchase one of disposable phones as part of the hospitals infection control policy."[8] This is because of an unseen fear that AIDS may spread through telephones.

Here is a real episode: when Rock Hudson was in a hospital dying from AIDS, Americans awfully worried about whether Linda Evans who kissed Rock Hudson on the television series "Dynasty" might contract the disease.[9] Much was aired on the 'Kiss' incident.

In another matter, the real-estate agents in California were instructed by their association to advise prospective home buyers about whether a house on the market had been owned by an AIDS patient, so that it may not be purchased.[10]

This was the bizarre scene in the very early years of the epidemic in none other than a highly advanced, civilized, and educated country, like United States of America. When the causative agent for AIDS was not clear, the mode of transmission of the disease was quite ambiguous, and consequently several misconceptions and myths ruled the society on AIDS. The researches that carried on AIDS cleared up many doubts and fears about the mode of transmission of this virus. Mere contact with the AIDS patient or mosquito bites cannot transmit the disease. However, if that is the situation in advanced countries, then one can imagine what would be the situation in the developing countries like India. Since the physician is a part of the public, he too had the influence of society's misconceptions and erroneous beliefs.

Man is a social being and he is greatly influenced by society. When society is facing a calamity, usually all the constituent institutions will be affected. The health care system, which is a part of the society, will have its influence, both positive and negative. In HIV/AIDS treatment, it is not totally the decision of the doctor alone, but very often; he/she may be influenced by their family members. In general, the physician had two responsibilities. On the one hand it is his moral responsibility to do justice to his profession, by extending his services to the sick and needy in accordance with the Hypocritic oath, and on the other hand he has to satisfy his family members and share their feelings and sentiments. The responsible physician is in a great dilemma, how to maintain a balance between both sides of the patient and the family in discharging his obligations to them. One may ask how the family comes into picture when a physician treats a HIV patient. Consider, for example the following incidents.

In mid 1980s, contrary to the hugging and handshaking of both the persons when they meet, which is a custom of the civilized western countries where those persons invariably touch each other, has been changed to the Indian custom of *namashkar*, where by joining both the palms, persons wish each other. Here touching the other person is avoided respectfully.

Similarly, family members of those doctors who are treating HIV positive patients may be developed some sort of psychological disturbance and unnecessary fear or phobia about contracting HIV by treating AIDS patients. A doctor may be skeptic in spite of he being a knowledgeable person. The health care providers stop treating HIV patients the moment they realize or know that they are attending on positive people is not correct. Indeed, it is a blessing to know about HIV status in advance. Consider, for instance, the following example.

If a person knows very well that he/she is going to deal with a poisonous snake in their garden, he will be more careful in each and every step. On the other hand, if he does not know that there is a poisonous snake in the garden, he will be usually careless in moving day and night or playing along with his children in the garden, and thus he may be a victim of a poisonous snake. Similarly, if the physician is not aware of the HIV status of the patient that he is treating, or if the surgeon is not aware of the HIV status of the patient on whom he is operating, or if an obstetrician is not aware of the HIV status of women to whom she is conducting delivery, then they are prone to accidental HIV infection, which is a professional hazard. If the health care personnel knew in advance about the HIV status of the treating patients, they take precautionary measures at each step of the treatment by following universal preventive guidelines. But unfortunately even today, 80% of the health care professionals are not convinced to treat enthusiastically HIV positive people. It may not be out of context to narrate several incidents of ill treating HIV positive people by medical personnel, which is not only a violation of human rights of the HIV positive persons, but also a violation of professional code of conduct.

Then, what about the code of conduct that has been formulated to the medical practitioners? Remarkably, such codes have been silent on the duty of physicians to treat patients in the times of epidemics. In the United States, the American Medical Association (AMA) code of 1847 was unique in its forthright assertion of such a responsibility. It says: "when any infectious disease that spreads quickly and kills a lot of people, it is their duty to face the danger and to continue their service for the alleviation of suffering, even at the risk of their own lives." This provision remained in the code until 1957, when a revised and shortened statement eliminated the stipulation saying that it is an old fashion. However, the era of epidemics has come to an end in the advanced industrial world.

But remaining in the code was a provision – first incorporated into the AMA's statement of professional responsibility of 1912, which in the absence of a strong assertion of a duty to care was to be a source of great confusion when AIDS confronted American society. "A physician shall, in the provision of appropriate patient care except in emergencies, be free to choose whom to serve". The AMA's Judicial Council has amended on professional freedom and ruled the refusals to treat on the basis of race, religion, or creed was unethical. In November 1987, in the seventh year of the AIDS epidemic, the council gave another ruling: "A physician may not ethically refuse to treat a patient whose condition is within the physician's current realm of competence, only because the patient is seropositive". By doing so, the AMA joined the American Nurses Association, which had a year earlier condemned discrimination against patients with AIDS.

Others have argued for a more universal obligation. But Physician and philosopher Edmund Pellegrino states: "To refuse to care for AIDS patients, even if the danger was greater than it is, amounts to decline something that is essential to being a physician."

The public health officials, who have stressed a universal obligation to treat, honestly may not directly face an HIV positive patient. However, the risk of HIV transmission is very much great. Does it require ethics of heroism to insist that every health care worker bear the responsibility of extending appropriate health care to the infected? Given the level of risk entailed in the face of HIV infection, even among surgeons and obstetricians, those who stress the obligation to treat argue that it was not heroism, but more straight forward duty that is essential. Doing duty without partiality by health care workers in case of HIV positive patients is a debatable issue to-day.

In nations that are poor and that can provide even the rudimentary health care services, several difficult ethical questions are emerging. No simple answers are possible in situations where so many pressing health care needs go unmet. The basic ethical obligation concerning with HIV persons is that they should not be discriminated.[11] A sick person is a sick person who needs attention whether the sickness is due to HIV or any another infectious disease.

William Haslett, in his book "Sketches and Essay" says: "Prejudice is the child of ignorance." The more the ignorance about AIDS, the more the prejudice about the HIV infected and affected. AIDS has awakened many sleeping giants in social terms. It has brought a new generation face to face with almost forgotten days of untreatable social contagion. Medical personnel must recognize a need for vigilance to combat this new social disaster and strictly avoid complacency.[12] It is true that all the physicians should sharpen their skills to mitigate the AIDS disaster.

The practice of medicine has traditionally been a paternalistic enterprise. In the past few decades, due to the influence of democratic principles in all walks of life, the medical profession also changed in its approach to physician–patient relationship. Now, there is public recognition of patients' rights, both morally and legally. This trend became universal.

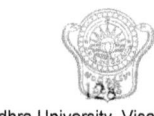

The American hospital association has promulgated a code of conduct to the health care providers, which is accepted by all hospitals in America. The rights of the patients, such as, the right to informed consent to treatment, the right to know one's diagnosis and prognosis, and the right to refuse treatment, even if it is life sustaining treatment. In case of competent patients, these rights may not be overridden even if a professional perceives to be in the best interests of the patient.

In Indian context due to factors like illiteracy and ignorance, the patient's right, are still questionable. However, informed consent for HIV testing and treatment are coming into vogue. It should be a real informed consent and not implied consent.

Refusing to treat an AIDS patient is illegal under the anti discrimination law. A doctor, who unlawfully terminates 'a doctor-patient relationship', may be liable in malpractice for abandonment. When that doctor is employed by a hospital, the hospital can be held vicariously liable for the actions of the doctor, and also for actions of other staff of the hospital, such as nurses and attendants. But in India many leading hospitals are failing to comply with the norms of medical practice.

A doctor or a hospital is required to exercise a reasonable degree of care and skill throughout the management of a patient. This includes diagnosis, treatment and follow-up of the patient. The standards expected from a professional are higher than that of an average individual. An action might be brought to recover damages as a result of negligent counseling after a positive HIV test result.[13] This is common in most of the western countries.

In India, the HIV positive patients are refused to admit in many hospitals both in government and in private sector. Several times the national news papers reported the matter: "All India Institute of Medical Sciences (AIIMS) which is a super specialty hospital in government sector, refused to treat HIV positive patients. If it is so, what would be the fate of HIV infected patients? Is it not violation of right of an AIDS patient to get proper treatment for his disease? After all, AIDS patients are also human beings, and to refuse treatment to them in hospitals is not only a violation of their rights but also it is morally objectionable to refuse treatment to them. Even after 28 years of war against AIDS, and in spite of many awareness campaigns, still many sections of population are ignorant about AIDS and its ramifications, and they are not getting proper treatment by admitting in hospitals where the specialist doctors are available to treat them.

Advertisements for AIDS Treatment and Unethical Practices:

Advertisements of drugs or magical cures for certain diseases such as AIDS, cancer, etc. should be banned, because they are misleading people suffering from such serious diseases. A controversy erupted in the year 2006 when the Ministry of Health, Government of India, sent a notice to the Yoga *guru* (teacher) Baba Ramdev questioning his claim to cure cancer and HIV/AIDS by the practice of Yoga. Such type of acts, require stringent laws to curb deceptive advertisements promising to cure through allopathy or alternate system of medicine. The Union health Ministry's move to ban advertisements concerning such treatments under the drugs and magical remedies act is a welcoming feature. Several quacks not only in India, even in the Western countries started claiming great deal of things up to an extent of making HIV positive to negative. Some other quacks are throwing net on innocent people, that is, offering treatments and magic-cures through internet, charging heavily and collecting fees via credit cards.

To deceive the HIV positive people and looting their money in huge quantities is an unethical practice, which is scandalous and disgraceful. It is regrettable that the government's soft approach on this issue becomes a source of strength to the people who are practicing homeopathy, allopathy, naturopathy and other systems of medicine, and some of these medical Practitioners are cheating the AIDS patients and their family members who are in great sorrow and distress. The innocent people who are in anxiety to find some cure to the AIDS are attracted by the deceptive advertisements seen in print and electronic media, but they never bothered about the bonafides of these claims. A Kerala State based company called 'Fair Pharma' used to give full back page advertisement in one of the Nation's leading weeklies 'India Today' with a claim that their medicine turns HIV positive people into HIV negative, which is an utter false, fake, and bogus statement. Cheating people in the name of AIDS treatment by several unqualified and fake doctors becomes order of the day all over the world.

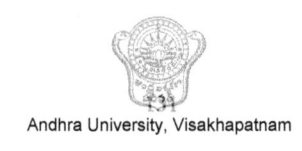

HIV Positive Health Care Persons (H.C.Ps):

The General Medical Council (GMC) advises all the doctors and health care providers to provide treatment to HIV positive patients and maintain confidentiality for which they are entitled. However, if there is a good reason to believe that the HCP is practicing or has practiced in a way which places the patients at risk, the HCP concerned must be advised before such information is passed on to an employer or regulatory body. The public interest disclosure act (1998) protects any member of the staff who discloses concerns about a colleague in the best interest of the public.[14] In case of HIV the same law is applied in India also.

Health Care Professionals and HIV Risk:

Epidemiologic studies show that needle stick injuries occur commonly to health care professionals, especially to the surgeons performing invasive procedure, and inexperienced hospital house staff and medical students. Efforts to reduce needle stick injury should focus on avoiding recapping needles and to use of safety needles whenever doing invasive procedures under controlled circumstances. The risk of HIV transmission from a needle stick with blood from an HIV infected patient is about 1:300. The risk is higher with deep punctures, large inoculate and source patient with high viral loads. The risk from mucous membrane contact is quantitatively too low.

Health care professionals who sustain needle stick injuries should be counseled and offered HIV testing as soon as possible. HIV testing is done to establish a negative baseline for workers' compensation claims in case there is a subsequent conversion. Follow-up testing is usually performed at 6 weeks, 3 months and 6 months.

A case control study by the (CDC) Center for Disease Control indicates that administration of Zidovudine following a needle stick injury decreases the rate of HIV seroconversion by 79%. Therefore, health care providers should be offered therapy with Combivir (Zidovudine 300 mg plus Lamivudine 150 mg orally twice daily) for 28 days. Health care providers who have exposed to persons who are likely to have anti-retroviral drug resistance (E.g. persons receiving therapy who have detectable viral loads) should be given individualized therapy, using at least two drugs to which the source is unlikely to be resistant. Some clinicians recommend triple combination regimens including a protease inhibitor for all occupational exposures, because of uncertainty about drug resistance. Others reserve these aggressive regimens for the higher risk exposures. Since reports have notified hepototoxicity due to Neverapini in this setting, this agent may be avoided. Therapy should be started as soon as possible after exposure and continued for 4 weeks. Unfortunately, there have been documented cases of seroconversion following potential parenteral exposure to HIV despite prompt use of Zidovudine prophylaxis. Counseling of the provider should include 'safe sex' guidelines, as prevention strategy.[15]

WHO Study on Safety of Injections:

The World Health Organization estimates that of the 1,200 crore (billions) to 1600 crore (billion) injections administered in the world every year, at least 50 percent are unsafe, particularly in the developing countries. While 82.7 percent of injections in India are administered for curative reasons, 17.5 percent are for vaccination. In Government Health establishment 68.7 percent injections were unsafe and 59.9 percent were dangerous in private clinics and hospitals.

The study classifies an injection as unsafe if it has the potential to transmit blood-borne viruses and/or it is administered faultily, which can cause local infection and/or reaction. The study found 53.1 percent injections dangerous because of faulty technique and 73 percent of them were unsafe because of the use of glass syringe. This made 62.9 percent of the injections unsafe.

The rural sector accounted for a higher 65.9 percentage of unsafe injections compared to urban areas, 54.9%. The safety is higher with plastic disposable syringes. The odds of an injection being unsafe are 12 times higher with glass syringes. Written guidelines for sterilization are available at only 10.1 percent of all health facilities in the country. Over half of the doctors and those who prescribe injections do not know the correct sterilization process. Only 84.2 percent of the government health facilities have sterilization equipment. Only 76.9 percent of immunization centers and 57.7 percent of private clinics use sterilization equipment. Only three fourths or 75.9 percent of the available sterilization equipment is functional.[16] Under this back ground, the hidden danger of trasmition of HIV through unsterile needles and syringes is alarming.

Hence, it looks to my mind that HIV/AIDS awareness special programmes have to be conducted to the hospital administration, doctors, nursing staff, and Para medical staff so that they collectively respond to the AIDS epidemics. In the emerging challenges of social, ethical and medical management of AIDS patients, the rights of patients, the rights of doctors, and the prerogative of hospitals have been creating moral dilemmas. Changing scenario of HIV/AIDS should solve the perplexity, the complexity and the magnitude of the problem. As a whole the AIDS infection presents a frightful challenge to the newly organized field of medical ethics and contemporary moral issues.

To sum up, in many countries the health care practitioners in general have not proven better informed or more enlightened than members of the lay public about the source and spread of HIV infection. Therefore, they too have shared the dysfunctional misperceptions and negative stereotypes that prevail among the general population, which resulted in refusal by some practitioners to treat the HIV infected. Disregard of the ethical duty to treat the sick gives rise to legal liability in different circumstances.[17]

Practitioners who decline to accept patients on the grounds of their actual or presumed HIV infection may be in breach of laws. Action may be initiated by persons denied services, but alternatively they may complain to police or other public authorities.

Health care practitioners who are members of professional associations whose ethical codes require non-discrimination, and / or who are licensed to practice subject to their observance of a code of professional practice, may face expulsion, and loss or suspension of license, and may violate contractual obligations of employment that require them compliance with ethical codes and rules of licensee. Thus both public law and private law may be applied against discriminatory conduct.

The legal measures outlined above enforce the duty to treat persons who are HIV infected. As per the law, refusal to treat due to the fear of HIV infection amounts to discrimination on grounds of physical or mental disability.

Some HIV positives may require medical care, for conditions not related to infection, or to illness they might have. For instance, in cases of HIV patients with limb fractures in accidents or pregnant woman preparing for child birth require treatment. The denial of services to them on account of their HIV status is illegal and discriminatory.[18]

Therefore, the physician's role has become so delicate with the entry of AIDS into the medical field. AIDS patients are posing risk like a double edged knife to physicians.

Can a health care provider or physician ethically reject a patient because of inability to pay or fail to pay the fee what they demand? The answer is both yes and no. While ethically the physician has wide latitude in selecting patients, there is less freedom in dropping a patient. Both legally and ethically, a physician is guilty of abandonment.

Of course, there are good reasons for terminating the relationship with a patient. However, termination of treatment requires that the physician should provide continuity of care by handing the patient over to another qualified professional.

The appearance of AIDS has raised old questions about the right of health care professionals to refuse treatment to a patient because of danger to themselves. Two points need to be considered in answering the question. First, all the rules of proportionality will apply. Secondly, because the professional has proficiency to serve society and the sick, the risks of harm must outweigh that professional obligation. In short, it takes more than normal risk to excuse health care professionals because of danger to them.

In the case of AIDS, all current research indicates that the risk of a health care professional to be infected by a patient is very small if proper procedures and universal precautions are followed. There is no danger if the health care professional with open cuts or breaks in exposed skin avoids working with the AIDS patient until the cuts and cracks are healed. These are temporary ethical excuses for not working with AIDS patients. On the other hand, a refusal based on dislike of homosexuals or drug users appears contrary to whole spirit of the health care profession.[19]

Economic Factors Involved in AIDS Treatment:

In the treatment of AIDS, very often the choice is not given to the patient whether he or she can afford it or not. A disease by itself has no discrimination or partiality towards poor and rich patients. Therefore, when treating a patient the physician recommends what is essential to the patient to save his life, irrespective of his economic condition or financial burden on him. In case of AIDS, since it is a new disease, many ARV drugs are not freely available and laboratory tests are also not within the reach of middle class or poor patients in India. Hence, the patients feel that the physician is prescribing expensive treatment which is a great burden to afford.

From the standpoint of ethics, prescribing expensive treatment to unaffordable people amounts to some sort of malpractice on the part of the doctor. The patients and the public think that by prescribing costly drugs, the doctor may be getting some commission from the pharmaceutical companies. This practice of prescribing costly drugs and expensive laboratory tests to the poor patients is linked with unethical practices in medical profession. In fact, the AIDS drugs and HIV tests are very costly. Hence, even a genuine physician who prescribes such tests and medicines is considered as torturing the poor patients.

As a physician, my personal sympathies are always with poor HIV patients. Some patients used to say, when we are going to die why we should waste money on treatment. The money we spend on treatment may be helpful for our children's education or marriage etc. But the truth is some what different. As a result of advanced researches in AIDS treatment, now the patients can be given a substantial life, and the death can be postponed dramatically. Thus, the physicians specialized in AIDS management are in great ethical dilemma what to do with poor patients. Without prescribing the essential costly tests, treating AIDS cannot be possible. On the contrary, prescribing costly tests and drugs to the poor patients who are unable to bear, suffer from psychological death. In such a situation, it is very difficult to decide, what is right and legitimate? Not prescribing the required costly tests and medicines means, allowing the patient to die prematurely. By counseling the patient, and preparing them to use the required costly drugs and treating them to live longer is the duty of the physician so that they can support their family. These are the pertinent moral issues that screw the brain of a physician. A private medical establishment, with commercial motto may not do free service to the AIDS patients, and the government AIDS care centers are not able to satisfy their clients.

HIV Infection and the Doctor-Patient Relationship:

In the treatment of AIDS, the doctor-patient relationship is founded on mutual trust. The exchange of information between doctor and patient should be based on honesty, openness and understanding of things in a proper perspective.

The General Medical Council has been impressed by the significant increase in the understanding of AIDS and AIDS-related conditions, both within the profession and by the general public. Many doctors are now prepared to regard these conditions as similar in principle to other infections and life-threatening conditions, and are willing to apply established principles in approaching their diagnosis and management. The Council believes that an approach of this kind will help doctors to resolve many of the difficulties which have arisen hitherto.

In the light of the general guidance, the Council has formulated the following instructions in relation to HIV infection and the conditions related to it.

Doctor's Duty towards Patients:

The Council expects that doctors will extend to patients who are HIV positive or are suffering from AIDS the same high standard of medical care and support, which they would offer to any other patient. It has, however, expressed its serious concern on reports where doctors have refused to provide HIV patients with necessary care and treatment. This culture, at times, reported in several Corporate Hospitals and private nursing homes in India.

It is improper for a doctor who lacks the necessary knowledge, skill or facilities to provide appropriate investigation or treatment for a patient and it is his duty that he should refer the patient to a professional colleague. However, it is unethical for a registered medical practitioner to refuse treatment or investigation for which there are appropriate facilities, on the ground that the patient suffers, from a condition which could expose the doctor to personal health risk. It is equally unethical for a doctor to withhold treatment to any patient on the basis of moral judgment that the patient's activities or lifestyle might have contributed to the ailment. Unethical behaviour of this kind may raise a question of serious professional misconduct. Even if few doctors exhibit such behaviour, it brings defame to the entire medical community.

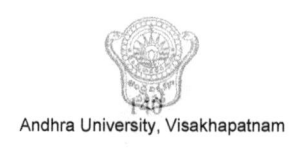

Duties of Doctors Infected with the Virus:

Considerable public anxiety has been aroused with reference to the HIV positive doctors, who are endanger to their patients. In such cases, the risk is very small and till today there is only one known case in the entire world, where HIV has been transmitted from a health care worker to his patients, in the case of dental treatment. Nonetheless, it is imperative, both in the public interest and on ethical grounds, that any doctor who is infected with HIV should seek appropriate testing and if found positive, must have regular medical supervision. This is not only for the welfare of the physician but also for the safety of the patients who are under his care.

Doctors who are HIV positive should also seek specialist advice on the extent to which they should limit their practice in order to protect their patients. Doctors must act upon that advice, which in some circumstances, would include a requirement not to practice or to limit their practice in certain ways. No doctor should continue in clinical practice merely on the basis of his own assessment of the risk to patients. The principles underlying this advice are already familiar to the profession, which has well-established policies and procedures designed to prevent the transmission of infection from doctors to patients.

It is unethical for doctors infected with HIV to put patients at risk by failing to seek appropriate measures. If such behaviour is found the Medical Council may restrict or remove the doctor's registration if necessary to protect the patient's health. This rule is not in force in

India. In the larger interest of the society this rule must be implemented in India. The Council has already given guidance on doctor's duty to inform an appropriate person or authority about a colleague whose professional conduct or fitness to practice may be called into question.

A doctor who knows that health care worker is infected with HIV and is aware that the person has not sought or followed advice to modify his or her professional practice, has a duty to inform the appropriate regulatory body or an appropriate person, who will usually be the most senior doctor. This methodology will minimize trauma to the doctor infected and consequences there after.

Rights of Doctors Infected with the Virus:

Doctors who were infected with the virus are entitled to expect the confidentiality and support afforded to other patients. Only in the most exceptional circumstances, where the release of a doctor's name is essential for the protection of patients, may a doctor's HIV status be disclosed without his or her consent. Many times doctors who were seropositive in India left the country to keep up their secrecy. It is another form of self imposed confidentiality.

Consent to Investigation or Treatment:

It has been long accepted, and is well understood within the profession, that a doctor should treat a patient only on the basis of the patient's informed consent. Doctors are expected in all normal circumstances to be sure to have their patient's consent to carry out investigative procedures or invasive techniques. As the expectations of patients increase, it is essential that both doctor and patient feel free to exchange information before investigation or treatment is undertaken.

This consent either verbal or written should be taken after due explanation in the language that is understood by the patient, and then only the procedure or treatment or investigation is to be done. In India due to various reasons this procedure is not being followed strictly. If it is verbal consent, a relative or friend's (third party) evidence is essential.

Testing for HIV: The Need to Obtain Consent:

The Council believes that all the general principles should apply for testing HIV infection, not because the condition is different from other infections, but because of the possible serious social and financial consequences involved in the testing. These problems would be better resolved by developing a spirit of tolerance rather than by medical action, but they do raise a particular ethical dilemma for the doctor in connection with the diagnosis of HIV infection or AIDS. The above factors provide a strong case for each patient to be given the opportunity, in advance, to consider the implication of submitting to such a test and deciding to accept or decline it.

Where blood samples are taken for screening purpose, as in antenatal clinics, there will usually be no reason to suspect HIV infection but even so the test should be carried out only where the patient has given explicit consent. Similarly, those handling blood samples in laboratories, either for specific investigation or for the purpose of research, should test for the presence of HIV only when they have given explicit consent. However in the most exceptional circumstances, where a test is imperative in order to secure the safety of persons other than the patient, and where it is not possible to obtain the prior consent of the patient, then testing without explicit consent is justified.

A particular difficulty arises in cases where it may be desirable to test a child for HIV infection. In such cases, the consent of a parent, or a guardian would normally be sought. However, in case the parent is not willing to come forward due to his own reasons, the doctor must first judge whether the child is competent to give consent to the test. If the child is judged competent to give his consent, then the doctor can be sought consent from the child. On the other hand, if the child is judged unable to give consent, the doctor must decide whether the interests of the child should over-ride the wishes of the parent. It is the view of the Council that it would not be unethical for a doctor to perform such a test without parental consent, provided that the doctor is able to justify that action is being taken in the best interests of the child.

AIDS Treatment and Confidentiality:

Doctors are familiar with the need to make judgments about whether to disclose confidential information in particular circumstances, and the need to justify their action for such a disclosure. The Council believes that, where HIV infection or AIDS has been diagnosed, the difficulties concerning confidentiality which arise will usually be overcome if doctors are prepared to discuss openly and honestly with patients the implication of their condition, the need to secure the safety of others, and the importance for continuing medical care of ensuring that those who will be involved in their care know the nature of their condition and the particular needs which they will have. The Council takes the view that any doctor who discovers that a patient is HIV positive or suffering from AIDS has a duty to discuss these matters fully with the patient.

When a patient is seen by a specialist who made diagnoses of HIV infection or AIDS, then the specialist should explain to the patient that the general practitioner involved in the patient's care can not be expected to provide adequate clinical management and care without full knowledge of the patient's condition. The Council believes that a majority of patients will readily accept to reveal their diagnosis to the treating general practitioners.

If the patient refuses to give his consent to the treating practitioner, then the specialist has two obligations to consider — the obligation to the patient to maintain confidentiality, and the obligation to other care givers whose own health may be put at risk. In such circumstances, the patient should be counseled about the possible consequences of his infection to the health care team. If the patient still refuses to allow the general practitioner to be informed, then the patient's request for privacy should be respected. The only exception to that general principle arises where the doctor judges the failure to disclose would put the health of any member of the health care team at serious risk. The Council believes that, in such a situation, it would not be improper to disclose such information. In the present circumstances, the need for such a decision arises very rarely, and even if it is needed, the doctor must be able to justify his or her action.

Similar principles apply to the sharing of confidential information between specialists or with other health care professionals such as nurses, laboratory technicians and dentists. All persons receiving such information must of course consider themselves under the same general obligation of confidentiality as the doctor principally responsible for the patient's care.

Doctor's Moral Obligation to Inform the Patient's Spouse:

Questions of conflicting obligations also arise when a doctor is faced with the decision, whether the patient's condition of HIV positive or suffering from AIDS should be disclosed to a third party, other than health care professionals, without the consent of the patient. The Council has arrived to the view that there are grounds for such a disclosure only where there is a serious and identifiable risk to an individual, who if not informed, would be exposed to infection. Therefore, when a person is found to be infected in this way, the doctor must discuss with the patient the question of informing to his spouse or other sexual partner. The Council believes that many patients will agree to disclose the information, but where such consent is withheld the doctor may consider it as his duty to inform the sexual partner in order to safeguard the persons from possible fatal infection. In reality, it is not happening in many Indian families. Doctors treating the HIV positives are not given the opportunity to inform the patient's spouse

.And many husbands are not informing their positive status to their wives or sexual partners. It is highly immoral and unethical to have sexual intercourse with a partner by concealing his or her HIV status.

Summary:

It is emphasized that the guidelines set out by the General Medical Council are intended to guide doctors in approaching the complex questions, which may arise in the context of HIV infection. It is not in any sense a code, and individual doctors must always be prepared, as a matter of good medical practice, to make their own judgments of the appropriate course of action to be followed in specific circumstances, and able to justify the decisions they make. The council believes that, in general, the doctors have acted compassionately, responsibly, and in a well informed manner in tackling especially the sensitive problems relating to the spread of HIV. In India similar guidelines have been formulated by NACO (National AIDS Control Organization) to safeguard the rights of the HIV positive persons. But their implementation is doubtful because regularly many disturbing reports are appearing in the press about the ill treatment of HIV/AIDS patients by some doctors and hospitals.

References:

1. J. Arras, *"The Fragile Web of Professional Responsibility: AIDS and the Duty to Treat"*. Hastings Center report 1988. Special supplement, April-May, 1988.

2. Zuger A and Miles SH, *"Physicians, AIDS and Occupational Risk: Historic Traditional and Ethical Obligations"*. Journal of the American Medical Association 1987; 258; pp.1924-28.

3. Usha K Baveja *"Legal and Ethical issues of HIV/AIDS: Diagnosis and management of HIV/AIDS, A Clinician's Perspectives"* (New Delhi, BI publications Pvt. Ltd.), pp.406-407

4. Fox D. *"The politics of physicians' responsibility in epidemics: a note on history"*, Hastings Center Report, Special Supplement, April-May, 1988.

5. Paul Volberding, M.D., and Donald Abrams, M.D., *"Clinical Care and Research in AIDS,"* Hastings Center Report (Aug 1985), p.16.

6. Raleigh, N.C *"The News and Observer"*, June 15, 1986.

7. William Check, *"Public education on AIDS: not only the medias responsibility"*, Hastings center report Aug., 1985, p.31.

8. "The Advocate," August 5, 1986.

9. The Rock Hudson Story, Part II, *"People"*, June 16, 1986, pp. 95-96.

10. The New York Times, June 26, 1985.

11. D.C. Jayasuriya, (ed), *"HIV law ethics and human rights"* First Edition: December 1995, pp 288-290.

12. S. Mukherjee, *"AIDS and the Physician"* in *"Medicine Update"*, by PM Dalal (ed), 1991, p.306.

13. Hall M.A and Ellman I.M, *"Health Care Law & Ethics in a Nutshell"*, (Minnesota: West Publishing Company, 1990).

14. Richard Pattman (ed), *"Ethical and Medico Legal Issues"*, Oxford Handbook of Genitourinary Medicine, HIV and AIDS, (New York, Oxford Medical Publications, 2007, p.34.

15. Mitchell H-Katz and Harry Hollander, (PG 1289) *"HIV INFECTION"* www.cmdthinks.com

16. The Hindu, Sunday, September 18, 2005.

17. Verkuyl D.A.A., *"Practicing Obstetrics and Gynecology in areas with a high prevalence of HIV infection"* Lancet 1995; 346, pp.293-96.

18. D.C. Jayasuriya (ed), *"HIV law ethics and human rights"* – Text and Materials, pp.79-80.

19. Thomas M. Garrett, Harold W Baillie, and Rosellen M. Garrett, *"Health Care Ethics - Principles and Problems"* pp. 67-68.

@@@@@

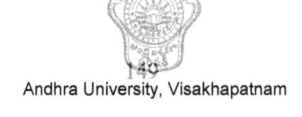

Chapter Six

AIDS Stigma and Discrimination: Ethical Confrontations

CHAPTER – VI

AIDS STIGMA AND DISCRIMINATION: ETHICAL CONFRONTATIONS

In any society, the stigma has two pronged influences on the people. In case of AIDS, AIDS infected and AIDS affected have been struggling a lot with stigma and discrimination in their day to day life. Even the AIDS service providers, such as, clinicians laboratory personnel, paramedical staff, nursing staff, the non-governmental organizations working in AIDS sector do face a considerable stigma and discrimination. It is a strange experience to reveal that the health minister belonging to one of the South Indian states expressed his resentment to talk to the social workers who are working in an AIDS service organization, might be due to fear of stigma or infection. In another incident, a MLA from another state in India was embarrassed to shake hands with the people working in HIV/AIDS clinics or HIV/AIDS voluntary organizations. He might have thought that by touching those people he may be infected.

The above two incidents were narrated by two Members of Parliament during Youth Parliament session on AIDS, which was inaugurated by the Honorable Prime Minister of India in New Delhi in November 2004. As I happened to be one of the speakers in the youth parliament, I could witness this bitter truth. These two incidents show the intensity of stigma attached to AIDS, and the resulting discrimination of people in the society. What should be the solution for such a dreadful dragon of stigma? Day by day the stigma attached to the AIDS, is killing more people than the AIDS itself. It is not only devastating many families but also ruining the human relations and sentiments. Many dedicated nursing staff and clinicians are in a moral dilemma, whether to continue to suffer with the stigma and humiliations attached to AIDS by attending on HIV positive people or deliberately avoid attending on HIV positive people. It is a very difficult problem to solve. Every sphere of human activity, such as, medical, educational, legal and political is being affected by AIDS epidemic. Due to fear of stigma and to avoid persons known to them, many HIV positive people are neglecting to take treatment or they prefer to go to far off places, to avoid their identity. Further, the positive patients avoid going to popular AIDS clinics like YRG care Chennai, APSAC clinics in Andhra Pradesh, RUBY Clinic in Pune or Surya Clinic in Visakhapatnam, because their identity may be known to others. Even if they come, they feel as though they are sitting on the thorns all the time they stay in the clinic.

By and large, the stigma attached to HIV/AIDS at the social, psychological, and cultural levels is dictating terms and conditions to the so called mighty man, how he has to behave and how he has to lead his future life journey. Poverty and ignorance are further crippling the HIV positive people. In early 1960s, when leprosy disease was so rampant, the Denmark Leprosy Trust was extensively working in India. Whenever the health care workers of the Denmark Trust visit any house in a village, the people around that house used to murmur among themselves, "Perhaps somebody in the house is having leprosy". Even the health care worker when walking in the street, people used to glare at him to which house he enters, and such is the intensity of stigma attached to leprosy in those days. The same scene is being repeated in a sharper way in the case of AIDS. In 1987, when I was in Britain, I visited an AIDS care ward in Manchester infirmary. Out of my curiosity, I requested the staff nurse working there to show me an AIDS patient. Then the two nurses on duty at that time, in all silence with glaring eyes and in a murmuring voice showed me the ward and told me the bed number without even looking at that side. I cannot forget that scene and the unique experience that I had, pasteurizing the very frightened nature of stigma or fear attached to AIDS, especially in a country like Britain, with an advanced knowledge, skills and scientific attitude.

Not much progress has been made during last two and half decades as far as minimizing the stigma attached to HIV/AIDS. If we consider the life experiences of Ms. Swaty and many other victims, we can understand how AIDS victims have been subjected to discrimination in the society.

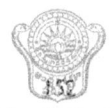

Swaty, the president of "HIV positive network" working in Medak district says: "I am living with HIV for the past eight years. When I first launched the network of HIV positive people, very few people came forward. But now, our network in the state has grown up to 60,000 people living with HIV. This is increasing day by day with large number of positive people joining the network and feeling comfortable. This solidarity will strengthen the network as a whole, and the voice of the positive people can be heard in national and international platforms to fight for the basic rights of people in the network. Swaty lamented that there are several cases of discrimination, especially legal discrimination against HIV positive persons. "People with HIV are denied their right to property also", she said.

In one case, the in-laws refused property rights to a woman and her kids, thinking that they will die with the AIDS disease and there is no need to give any property to them. This tendency among people is the main reason for not spending even a small amount of money on HIV positive persons thinking that it is waste to spend on those persons who are going to die. This is a misconception, because many positive people are leading long and quality life with the advent of modern drugs. If proper treatment is given HIV/AIDS patients also can live longer and lead almost a normal life like any other patient suffering from asthma, or diabetes mellitus, or psoriasis.

Another woman, Mayuri, was deserted by her husband after she was tested HIV positive. She said: "Three years ago, I was tested HIV positive. We have one son. My husband took away him. In that desperate situation, I have been attempted to suicide in 2005, and I was taken to a hospital by my friends where I was counseled. Then, I came out of the shock and became normal and developed a positive attitude to my life. "Now I am helping others, but my husband is seeking divorce."

People living with HIV have been facing many social and moral problems in their day to day work, ranging from difficulty in getting work to live or getting government pensions or to educate children due to stigma.

Ramya, who is a HIV positive, says: "I am from Guntur town and my husband died of AIDS, and I came to Hyderabad as I was facing serious discrimination in my native town. Although, I produced the death certificate of my husband for widow pension in Hyderabad, the authorities insisted that I should get the pension in my home town Guntur only, which I deserted for my dignity and self-respect." This type of attitude of government officials towards pensioners like me is so painful.

ART centers in the state have been providing medication for AIDS related illness, but nutritional care is not provided to the patients. Though some NGOs provide nutritional support, they cover only 30 to 40% of the persons living with HIV. As the treatment and investigations are costly, some organizations working for HIV positive people are demanding the Andhra Pradesh government to extend the Arogyasri scheme (a government sponsored free medical treatment) to cover HIV positive cases also. If the government includes AIDS in the

Arogyasri scheme, then it will be a great relief to thousands of HIV/AIDS victims.

In the year 1998, around 11.30 A.M., when I was in my clinic, a woman aged about 58 years in deep anguish entered my chamber, pushing away the heavy crowd of patients. I politely offered her a seat and enquired about the reason for her anxiety, tension, and impatience. Without listening to me, in utter distress, she broke into tears and asked me in a shivering voice, "Doctor please give me a medicine to die". Then, I asked her in eagerness, Why you have decided to die? Then I told her, I am here to save lives but not to give medicine to kill my patients. But she least listened to me and continued demanding the medicine to die. Meanwhile her husband, who was standing behind joined her. Then, I tried my level best to console her. After some time, she cooled down, and again she cried loudly without bothering her surroundings and told me that she had only one son, who has a boy aged about three years and who is the beloved grandson of this woman. Her daughter-in-law is not allowing this grandmother to touch her grandson, because this poor old lady turned HIV positive in a pathetic incident.

A couple of years back, when she had a gynecological problem, she was examined by a gynecologist and was suggested hysterectomy (removal of uterus). This operation was conducted in a rural hospital where she was given blood transfusion during that surgery. Her husband brought the blood from his friend, a donor whose blood was given to her without testing for HIV. Even after three months, when the wound was not healing, she was thoroughly investigated, performing all kinds of blood tests including HIV test whose result came as positive. The woman at that old age became positive and she is not allowed to touch her grandson by her daughter in law, due to fear of infecting the child. Further, she was kept in a single room away from their house, and food is being thrown on her from a distance. Because of this discrimination and isolation of her from the rest of the family, and not allowing her to touch her grandson, she attempted twice to commit suicide. After having heard about me, she came all the way from Khammam town to enlighten herself of the hidden dangers of spreading the infection to her grandson by touching or hugging. On knowing her episode, I asked whereabouts of her daughter-in-law. The woman said that she was sitting in the car in front of our hospital. Then, I told her to bring her daughter-in-law to my chamber. She and her husband (son of this old woman) came to me. I clarified their doubts and fears on AIDS, and in order to dispel the myth that HIV spreads through contact or bodily touch, immediately I hugged that old lady in front of all of them, and explained to them that there is no point of unnecessary AIDS phobia. By any social contact such as hands shaking, hugging, social kiss, living together, sleeping on the same cot, using the same toilets/bathrooms there is not even an iota of risk of spreading the infection from positive people to normal people. This living instance narrates that how innocent women like this old lady are being wounded physically, psychologically, and socially due to hasty blood transfusions without proper scientific testing for HIV.

Safety of the blood in government and commercial blood banks is another big concern. The government should impose strict guidelines in undertaking Blood Transmissions and people who need blood should be doubly careful, otherwise HIV infection through blood transfusion is a lurking problem.

There are some encouraging stories of HIV positives. Some positive mothers have formed as "self-help groups" and are funding their own treatment and sharing their sorrows and pleasures. Nandini, a resident of Gachibowli, says: "we have formed a self-help group. Each member saves Rs.250/- per month and an NGO gives a matching grant of another Rs.250/-. This way we help each other in need". Like this the positive action groups are coming up to frontline in the recent past to fight stigma and discrimination attached to the AIDS.

In order to avoid discrimination, organizations like APSAC (Andhra Pradesh AIDS Control Society) started giving preference to appoint HIV positive people as out reach workers. However, many departments like fire, police, and navy are not recruiting HIV positive candidates because AIDS is a misunderstood malice. This attitude should be changed.

AIDS Stigma and Moral Confrontations:

Stigma is known to the world from days immemorial. It refers to the people's feelings of disapproval about a particular illness or certain ways of behaviour. The social stigma is attached to the diseases like leprosy, or mental illness, or HIV/AIDS. Also certain risk behaviour people such as homosexuals, bisexuals, and commercial sex workers, in particular, have been stigmatized by linking AIDS to their promiscuous conduct. A few years ago, the sex workers in Bangkok expressed heavy resentment on the use of word "commercial". They questioned why do people call us commercial sex workers? Why not people call professional doctors as commercial doctors, teachers as commercial teachers, and lawyers as commercial lawyers? They too do their profession for money just like us. Since then, many leading agencies stopped using the word commercial sex workers and started using only sex workers.

Regrettably, from the very beginning of the AIDS epidemic, certain groups only have been labeled as "risk" groups and they are being discriminated and treated in a cruel and inhuman way. The groups such as 'sex workers', 'homosexuals', 'truck drivers', 'sea men', 'IV drug users' and others became victims of such discrimination. It implies that these groups alone are the culprits of HIV/AIDS transmission. In reality, even general public can transmit the virus. Then, why some groups of people exclusively are stigmatized? On what grounds the risk behaviour is discriminated? Of course, a few of the truck drivers may be promiscuous. Is it morally right to blame the entire group of truck drivers? The same thing applies to other groups as well.

Some nationalities and ethnic groups have also been victimized. People of Haiti Island, some ethnic groups of African countries, and members of some gay clubs have been discriminated *suomotto*. In India, when 10 sex workers were first identified in Madras as HIV positives in 1986, the land cost there has come down drastically as if Madras (Chennai) is the harvesting place for AIDS. It is amazing to note that how negatively the consequences of AIDS will affect every sphere of social life, whether it may be business, or education, or industry. Further, despite a crystal clear evidence that the HIV/AIDS cannot be spread by casual contacts, children with HIV/AIDS, and even children born to HIV parents who were negative HIV status, have also been barred from schools. Several establishments have summarily dismissed their workers, insurance companies have refused coverage and tenants have been evicted from houses.[1] Giving punishment to a HIV person is against to the spirit of human rights, because most of the positives are active, healthy and productive. Refusing coverage by insurance companies for the positive people is unethical because the company has no respect for human life.

Legal restrictions on the movement of persons with HIV/AIDS have led to all forms of discriminatory treatment. Even after three decades of AIDS epidemic, Australia has imposed restrictions on entry of HIV positive people into their country. The United State of America allows entry of positive people with certain conditions, and many countries in the world do have objections for the entry of positive people into their respective countries. However, the entry restrictions are now and then liberalized due to agitations organized by AIDS activists. Some international companies, while recruiting work force for abroad services from India, vehemently object and cancel their appointment letters in case anyone found HIV positive in the selected list. It is really so pathetic, and it amounts to violation of human rights. The United Nations commission on human rights resolution on HIV/AIDS (resolution no.1995/44 adopted on 3rd March 1995) clearly says: "Recognizing the increasing challenges, presented by HIV/AIDS require, renewed efforts to ensure universal respect for an observance of human rights and fundamental freedom for all, as well as the avoidance of HIV/AIDS related discrimination and stigma."

But in practice, it is not being followed in toto, and even if it is followed by some people, it is merely for the sake of satisfying the rule. Hence, young HIV positive people have been facing hurdles at every stage, and those who are very sensitive are slowly going underground.

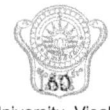

In this context, I wish to confess that I had an opportunity to address the United Nations General Assembly in June, 2008, which was attended by several world leaders including Bill Clinton. In one of the sessions, I have argued that why many countries are still discriminating positive people and not allowing them into their country. Secondly, it is inhuman to cancel appointments of the young positive asymptomatic and totally healthy individuals for simple reason of their being positive. My demand was that since many positive people can live with good health and enough energy to work for several years, say about 10 to 15 years, denying them employment is nothing but snatching away food from their mouths. This type of immoral attitude of corporate sector towards the young unemployed positive people further kills them psychologically, and deprives sustenance to them and their dependent family members.

On the other hand, if they are permitted to travel abroad and allowed to work comfortably, they will have redoubled vigour with reinforced self confidence to make use of their skills for the national development while helping themselves and their families. If once they are employed, their financial stand would definitely give them an opportunity to use continuously the high cost drugs of Highly Active Antiretroviral Therapy (HAART), in addition to intake of highly nutritious balanced diet. When I addressed on this issue with due respect, and raised my voice to safeguard the rights HIV positive people, huge number of delegates from all corners of the globe endorsed my demand and expressed their solidarity with thumping applause.

Imposing legal restrictions on freedom of internal travel due to compulsory hospitalization or quarantine or isolation is a violation of the right to freedom of movement. There are also restrictions on sexual behaviour. In other words they dictate or control the sexual behaviour of positive persons. Restrictions are imposed on donation of blood, semen, breast milk or organs, of course no positive individual donates blood or semen etc irresponsibly. Restrictions on freedom of occupation, so that positive people are controlled when they choose an occupation. Also there are miscellaneous forms of restrictions such as marriage contracts. Positive people are legally restricted in making marriage contracts among themselves. In less than a decade, a substantial number of restrictions have been emerged for application to persons with HIV/AIDS. Nevertheless not all of them are entirely new to the field of public health legislation. When we analyze these legal restrictions, they seem to be counter-productive rather than advantageous to restrict the spread of HIV. But we can profoundly say that these restrictions enhance badly the arena of stigma and discrimination. The HIV virus on one side and the human virus on the other are brutal, and are jointly firing against the human rights, human sentiments, the very sensitive layers of self-esteem, and eventually on the very existence of human race.

In many instances, these restrictions have been extended to cover HIV/AIDS disregarding the fact that these restrictions were not applicable to this disease. In fact, these restrictions are initially formulated to deal with the specific contagious or communicable diseases or conditions. Neither HIV nor AIDS fits into this label of a contagious or communicable disease or condition in the strict sense of the term. Even after 10 years of close monitoring, HIV is not known to have been transmitted through social contacts except through one of the three well documented modes through sex, through needle, through blood. In other words HIV virus transmits through infected needles, infected blood, from positive mother to child, and heterosexual or homosexual route while having sex with a positive person. These restrictions limit the rights and freedom of individuals with HIV/AIDS, even in the absence of definitive evidence that such restrictions are necessarily effective in slowing down HIV transmission. It is a great injustice, to tie the limbs of positive people by unnecessary restrictions, with an apprehension of possible spread of infection by them. This is an unethical and inhuman practice to put unreasonable restrictions on HIV/AIDS persons.

Discrimination against HIV/AIDS Persons:

Discrimination in the health care system still exists though some changes are gradually happening for the good of AIDS patients.

When a surgery is required to a positive person, then many government hospitals are creating problems to take up the case. Private hospitals do not treat HIV infected people readily. Even if they agree to admit and extend care and treatment, many hospitals are charging them exorbitantly.

Discrimination against HIV Positive Children:

Ms. Ruben recalled one of the many instances when Indian network of positive people (INP) had fought for the cause of students who were discriminated and denied admission to schools. "Basically the school authorities were ignorant of the disease and consequently they have apprehensions about HIV/AIDS and its spread to other students. But once they are made aware, children were admitted," she said. This is possible only in government run schools. In private schools, the administration was unwilling to admit positive children in spite of their awareness on AIDS. This sort of discrimination at the school level will badly injure the tender minds of the children.

Different Facets of Stigma:

Stigma stems from the way society links the person's positive status with his morality and moral behavior. "In the southern part of

India, HIV is linked to the person's sexual behaviour. Social stigma is the extreme if the infection is through sexual route, and it is less if it is through infected blood transfusion, IV drug use or other routes. So people usually say they got infected through infected blood transfusion or through unsterile needles while taking injection from a quack or rural medical practitioner, or through a contaminated blade at barber shop (saloon) and so on.

In the absence of a drug or vaccine, issues of individual liberty and functional effectiveness of coercive measures tend to loom large when measures such as detention, isolation and quarantine are considered. In those countries where AIDS has been included under existing classifications of communicable diseases, or sexually transmitted disease, it is possible to obtain help for all those measures, which curtail individual's liberty or restricting mobility or requiring submission of tests, and treatment. In some countries these measures extend even to the identification of sexual partners. In the United States, some states provide for both quarantine and isolation. Similar legal provisions exist in countries like China.[2] In Cuba HIV seropositive persons have been sent to a sanatorium located in a Havana suburb.[3]

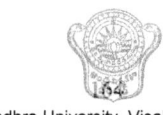

One argument is that such coercive and restrictive measures are counter productive and fortunately such measures are not practiced in India. The government is very considerate and never imposes stringent restrictions and it is trying to dispel such beliefs and restrictions with the help of NACO. Nonetheless the public attitude towards HIV positives is very painful and the following life sketches reveal the intensity of hardships that are faced by the HIV infected persons.

Bad Treatment of Hospital Staff:

Nancy, a HIV positive woman aged thirty years, was infected by her husband seven years ago. She says: "I came to know that I was HIV positive when I was pregnant. My second daughter was also HIV positive, At that time, I didn't know what AIDS was and the hospital staff scared me. The hospital attendant used to gossip about my disease with others. The nurse was throwing bred on me, and said to my mother that I would die soon. However, it took a lot of time for my family to accept me." Nancy continued, "I stay with my parents, but a separate cooking area and a separate toilet were allotted to me. I don't understand why people can't treat us on a par with tuberculosis, asthma, or cancer patients. I have now started working for children living with HIV. I monitor 27 children and take them for tests and support them with all their daily needs. This service to positive kids is giving me utmost satisfaction".

Refusal of Relatives:

Kamakshi, a 35 years old woman of Bhuvanagiri town got HIV infection nine years ago. She used to work as a sweeper, but was removed from service as she used to suffer frequently with fever, cough, diarrhoea etc. After ART treatment she recovered and now she works in a school as an attendant. "My husband is a rickshaw puller and he infected me. He himself died of AIDS", she told.

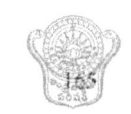

She narrates her difficulties as: "My daughter is studying in a private school. If they know about my condition, they will throw her out of the school. I am more worried about my daughter's education and her future: In fact, even my relatives don't allow me inside their house. When I visit them, I have to sit at the door to the entrance of the house. As soon as I leave they clean the place with Phenol. When I am thirsty my neighbors refuse to give me even a glass of drinking water. They close the doors soon they notice me. My life is miserable, but I am struggling daily to live in this cruel world only for the sake of my pretty daughter".

HIV/AIDS - Social Stigma and Discrimination:

Subhu tops his class, paints beautifully, and is full of zest for life. But no one can see the pain hidden behind this 11 year old innocent smile. He dreams to become a doctor despite knowing that he faces certainly death and that too for no fault of his. Subhu's parents Anamika and Aravind were tested positive when he was nine months old. Subhu was tested positive for HIV when he was 18 months old. For the fear of society, his father committed suicide leaving wife and lovely son. His mother Anamika has joined in an NGO and working as peer counselor, who is the only hope for him. Subhu was given antiretroviral therapy (ART) when he was just two years old and he is continuing the therapy and doing well.

The pain is more among children as they have to take several medicines to avoid various infections associated with the disease. Pills for HIV, Pills to control fever, Pills to control diarrhea, and pills to control cough, like this 15-20 tablets per day put the child and the parents or guardians in stress. If the parents are poor, purchasing all these tablets once again is a big burden.

The stigma associated with the disease makes things worse for children. If the school administration knows that a particular child is HIV positive, they keep the child to sit separately in the school or send him from the school. This type of negative attitude is further killing the children. Suraj is a ten year old boy, and he lost his father and sister because of AIDS. He was forced to change the school after parents of his classmates insisted that the school authorities should sent him from the school. Again, Suman another fourteen years old guy, who lost both his parents due to HIV, and he suffered a great deal due to the stigma and discrimination, from his neighbours, relatives and friends all the time. He goes to the ART centre regularly for treatment and started attending meetings of positive network.[4] The positive net works are functioning very effectively even in our country to safeguard the rights of people living with HIV/AIDS.

Mouli, an young man got shocked when he was diagnosed as HIV positive. For a few days, he thought that it was a death warrant to him. In the mean time, a friend referred him to Osmania General Hospital for counseling and treatment. Mouli got a new life there through a scientific counseling and proper treatment.

Raman, a 32 year old computer graduate and a resident of Secunderabad, is a confident man. He was helped to overcome the trauma by doctors, and motivated by a counselor at Integrated

Counseling and Testing Centre (ICTC). He is now able to lead a normal life and got married to a HIV positive network lady. After his marriage, with a sense of gratitude he says: "I am thankful to the team of doctors and supporting staff for enabling me to lead a happy marital life." Now with the advent of antiretroviral therapy (ART), and formation of network for people living with HIV/AIDS to tide over psychological problems faced by them, many positive people are quite happy and leading a normal life. The initiative taken by the Author and certain NGOs involved in HIV/AIDS care have made the difference. Today several ICTCs are operational in the country.

A young man by name Rushi belonging to the old town of Hyderabad was tested HIV positive in 2005. He got the treatment at a private hospital for sometime as his CD4 count fell down to 327 cells per cu.mm. He abandoned the therapy a month later, due to financial constraint and lack of knowledge that he has to take lifelong treatment. Two years later he suffered heavy weight loss and got opportunistic infections, such as diarrhoea, and oral thrush. After coming to know about the facilities available at government hospital, he visited the hospital and found his CD4 count was 150 cells per cu.mm. Doctors immediately gave him ART after counseling. He found the atmosphere and the support from the staff of the hospital was very inspiring. Six months later, his CD4 count increased to 600 cells per cu.mm. His trauma and agony thus came to an end. Later he advised all his friends, who were known for their high risk behaviour to visit ICTC

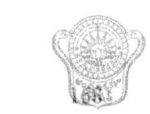

(Integrated Counseling and Testing Centre). He becomes a role model for others, and he turned as outreach worker for the community.[5]

In November, 1987 when I was in Manchester, UK, to attend an international conference, namely "Caring for AIDS", I happened to see an article in the London newspaper. That was a box item wherein a school girl, aged about 7 years was stoned by the public. The reason was that her mother was HIV positive. The demand from the parents of other school children was that the child's name should be removed from the school register. In India too, very often we see the similar news items demanding the school principal, not to admit HIV positive children to the school. In the case of the UK child, it was a pitiable scene where for no fault of the child, she is being stoned. She is not even a HIV positive, but her mother was. What sin this poor girl has committed for such inhuman treatment? When such an event happened in an advanced country like Britain, with high literacy, scientific outlook and rational thinking, what is the fate of Children belonging to HIV parents in a developing country like India? Therefore, as soon as I returned to India, I have launched a massive AIDS awareness campaign and addressed the press club of India, in Delhi in November 1987 informing the public and the professional colleagues about the preventive measures of HIV/AIDS.

A Young Woman with HIV Status Thrown Out of the House:

Komali, a young woman lost her husband and only son to AIDS. She is living with HIV and making all efforts to lead a normal life at Allahabad. She is, in fact, grateful to the health department and the

Allahabad Network for PLWHAs (People Living with HIV\AIDS) for making her aware about her rights.

Thrown out of the house by her relatives, Komali suffered a great depression, but she fought for her property rights to reclaim everything from her in-laws, which she and her husband had accumulated for themselves. Despite the reluctance of her in-laws to give her due share of a piece of land that was in the name of her husband, Komali fought a legal battle till she managed to get the land transferred in her name. Since she is bold and tenacious woman, she could win the case in the court of law. Scores of HIV positive widows who acquired the infection from their husbands are forced to lead their lives in distress. After the death of their husbands, most of them are disowned by their families or denied property rights. Unquestionably, there are many who live in despair due to lack of awareness about their rights. A bold woman like Komali, who learnt about the legal rights, claimed for what was legitimately belonging to her.

The secretary of Allahabad Network for People Living with HIV\AIDS (ANP+), claims that many HIV positive widows contact them to know about their rights. She added that HIV positive people too have fundamental rights, which should be uphold at all levels. ANP+, offers support to such women by educating them about their rights and even takes them to the government offices like DRDA (District Rural Development Agency), which offer assistance to these women. Hence these widows too can lead a normal life.

Many NGOs are working for HIV+ people with twin objectives of motivating them, who are suffering silently, and to fight for their rights, and make their voices heard to the authorities who plan welfare programmes for the benefit of such persons.

Sowmya's story too is similar to Komali. After getting married to a Banda-based person who worked in Mumbai as a labourer, she got infected with HIV. In fact, shortly after her marriage Sowmya learnt that her husband was HIV+ even before their marriage. After some time, her husband died and she found herself alone to fight for her rights. However, she got timely help from some health department officials who informed her about the property rights, and Sowmya claimed for her share of property from her in-laws.

Similar to these cases, many HIV infected people have horrifying tales to narrate. Several service organizations are offering all sorts of assistance to these people so that they can lead a normal life. Though governments have started various schemes for the welfare of such persons, they are not sufficient to meet the requirement of those people. Government of Andhra Pradesh has launched a pension scheme to HIV positive people and it is distributing double ration to the HIV positive children. APSRTC (Andhra Pradesh State Road Transport Corporation) is providing concessional fare to HIV positive person and one assistant to go to ART centers for treatment.[6]

With the support of NGOs and also some help from the Government, things are now moving better for HIV positive widows, who are assured of justice and a respectable life. While the government has already made free treatment available to HIV+ persons, they need a sustained mechanism for a comprehensive help. Many state Governments are supplying nutritious diet, free rice, and free grains to some extent. Indian Railways also offering free and concession fare to positive people and their attendents.

In the state of Gujarat, at Vododara, a family of four committed suicide on March 17, 2009. Mr. Deepak and Mrs. Pannaben are a couple suffering from AIDS. The couple gave poison to their two daughters and they also consumed it and committed suicide. Police investigation revealed that the couple was positive and was tired of long treatment, and finally all the family members committed suicide out of frustration.[7] This type of incidents is herd regularly from the media, in the era of AIDS. The other reason behind these suicides is the stigma associated with AIDS that is more horrifying.

Pasted on the Wall as Positive:

In an open violation of the guidelines of National AIDS Control Organization (NACO), the staff of the state-owned Swaroop Rani Nehru Hospital, a part of Motilal Nehru Medical College at Allahabadd, barely pasted an 'HIV' sign on the wall behind the bed of an AIDS patient and refused treatment to him. This sort of behaviour of medical staff is a shameful instance to the entire medical fraternity.

The HIV positive man from Pratappur block, with acute infection, was brought to the SRN hospital. The doctors initially refused to admit him, said the sources. They relented only after the Allahabad Network for People Living with HIV Positive (ANP Plus) took up the matter with the district magistrate and the hospital administration. However in the next morning, the staff wrote "HIV" on a piece of paper and pasted it on the wall behind patient's bed in surgical emergency ward. When the attendants of patient objected and reported the matter to ANP Plus, the sign was removed on the instruction of anti-retroviral Medical officer of SRN hospital. Meanwhile enough damage has been done to the patient and his family.

In spite of all these incidets, next day the staff of the hospital wrote ART (Anti-Retroviral Therapy) on the wall and tied a red ribbon, the monogram of NACO, on the IV (intra venous) drip stand, said the relatives of the patient. This is also another way of insult to the positive people. Usually the hospital, the nursing staff and the medical officers should know about the status of the patient to take universal precautions. This can be done confidentially by writing on the case sheet as 'NACO + Ve', which will help the attending staff to be more careful to prevent infection to themselves. It is the fundamental duty of the hospital staff to maintain confidentiality, but contrary to it they are discriminating HIV patients by advertising about them in the ward of the Hospital. Further, the doctors allegedly refused to treat the patient, saying proper medical kits were not available in the hospital. The attendants of the patient and the members of NGO reported the matter to District Magistrate and Chief Medical Officer.

"We were asked to purchase gloves and other items from outside. We also had to do the dressings of the patient," said the attendant. Due to this ill treatment and the antipathy of the hospital staff and doctors, the family got fed up and took discharge and went away. The Superintendent-in-Chief of SRN hospital said that she has ordered a departmental inquiry into the matter. She also said that she had provided five medical kits for the treatment of the patient. Not only the SRN Hospitals, even today 90% of Hospital in India are refusing the admissions of HIV positive people or ill treating the positive patients.

It is an offence to refuse treatment to an HIV positive patient and it is a more serious offence to advertise such and such person is HIV positive. The behaviour of doctors and hospital staff of SRN Hospital was uncalled for and strict action must be taken against those responsible for such actions.[8] The other argument is that rather than giving punishment, it may be suggested a scientific way of awareness on HIV/AIDS, clarifying all the doubts to medical staff that is helpful in long run.

Relatives Killed:

A 45-year-old farmer, his wife and son, were allegedly killed by their relatives after it was discovered that they had full-blown AIDS in Lucknow. Mr. Jimany a farmer, who has been sick for about two years went to Baba Raghav Das Medical College (BRDMC) in Gorakhpur where he was admitted for a complete medical check-up following complaints of chronic fever and acute weight loss. Under this background he was tested HIV positive in May 2007.

Jimany was prescribed medication spreading over six months. Despite taking the medicines regularly, his condition continued to deteriorate to the extent that he was rendered bed ridden in December

2007. Unable to meet the expenses incurred while he was in the hospital, he requested the doctors to discharge him but he regularly visited the BRDMC as an out-patient.

Meanwhile he suffered another jolt when his wife Chandrika too tested HIV positive in January 2008. The worst came for the family when their son too tested positive about a fortnight. Already he is under debt with no source of income, and finally Jimany visited the hospital in Gorakhpur on July 24, 2008 and returned home with hopelessness, and decided not to continue the medical treatment any more.

According to the report of Chandrika's father Sunder, Mr.Jimany and Mrs. Chandrika and their only son were treated as outcaste by his family members ,who feared that they would also catch the disease if they interact with them.

Eventually on Sunday morning, the three persons were murdered by Jimany's own brothers, and their bodies were cremated without informing even to the near and dear family members including Chandrika's parents. When Chandrika's family came to know about the incident, they lodged a complaint with the Chapiya police station of Gonda accusing Jimany's brothers of murdering the three, said the station officer. Additional superintendent of police (ASP) of Gonda Mr.Saroj, however, told that "during initial investigations the accused have claimed that Jimany and his family had committed suicide and that they simply went ahead with the cremation without informing any body. However, they failed to explain why they did not inform the police when three family members committed suicide at a time that requires, a thorough police investigation." ASP further added that since the bodies of the deceased have been cremated there was nothing which could help to establish the exact cause of deaths of victims.[9]

Obscene SMS to a Widow:

Despite the efforts are made by the government and non-governmental organizations (NGOs) not to stigmatize and look down the people living with HIV/AIDS, especially the women in Manipur, are being insulted by many well educated people. Nonetheless, several positive persons are able to live with a firm decision to fight the infection with the support of the government and non governmental authorities.

In July 2009, with the help of Lawyers Collective, a widow living with HIV/AIDS in Thoubal district lodged a complaint with the Chief Judicial Magistrate of Thoubal, against a graduated youth, alleging of hurting her modesty by sending SMS with obscene words and luring her to indulge in immoral activities.

In response to the complaint, a case was registered with the Thoubal police station under section 500 (deals with Punishment for defamation) and section 509 (Word, gesture or act intended to insult the modesty of a woman) and arrested the person. But in the later part, the woman withdrew the case. "When the person offered apology at my feet with a plea that he would not indulge in such activities in future, further urging me to forgive him for the sake of his prestige, I felt pity for him. The person admitted his misconduct and offered apology in the presence of elderly people. Hence, I decided to withdraw the case from the police", the widow said.

She further added: "if convicted in this case, the youth might be ordered for a two year jail imprisonment. But I wanted nothing else except the educated youth should realize what is good and what is bad. Besides I would not like to go to police station and court repeatedly in connection with the case, as I thought it is not good to appear in the court frequently for a woman like me who lost my husband and struggling for life with the dreaded disease."

Appreciating the decision of the woman, legal cum advocacy officer of the Lawyers' Collective said that the widow is a "double victim". How difficult the lonely life of a HIV/AIDS positive widow in the society is well known to all of us. Educated men must know it better. Secondly, it is an illegal act to try to demoralize a woman and hurting her modesty by using obscene words through mobile as mentioned in the section 509 of the Indian Penal Code (IPC). Despite all this, on humanitarian ground, the man has been forgiven by the woman in presence of elderly people. The efforts of the government and NGOs to control the dreaded disease will be useless, unless the society respects these victims. Lawyers' Collective tried its best to deliver justice to the woman without delay. Police and court also helped a lot in her case.[10]

HIV Stigma and Killing of Innocent People:

In a village in Chittoor district of Andhra Pradesh, India, when a person died of HIV/AIDS, his corpse was dragged like that of a dead dog in the streets of that village by his relatives. What an inhuman treatment it was. In the flood of social stigma, the human sentiments, affection between family members, and human values have been swept in the streets of that village. It shows how forceful the stigma is. A couple of years ago, in the state of Bihar, when people in a village came to know about a person's HIV condition, he was burnt alive in a cattle-shed. It shows how cruel and disrespectable are the people for human life. All fundamental human values have been null and void in the face of HIV/AIDS. No religion or scripture teaches to kill a person brutally by burning alive.

In another incident, when the people of a small town came to know that the owner of a small shop is HIV positive, they forcibly sent him to the outskirts of the town, isolated and banished him, besides people boycotting to purchase any provisions from his shop. The stigma attached to HIV/AIDS, and its accompanying discrimination and apprehensions is shaking the very foundations of the civil society and its ideals.

As the HIV stigma is spreading like a wild fire with multiple faces in the nuke and corner of the country with a greater speed than the HIV virus, the common man is scared of stigma attached to the AIDS, rather than AIDS disease itself. It is not an exaggeration to say that the 'stigma' is devastating many families with inhuman treatment and cruel deaths.

The Government, the corporate sector, the NGOs, and the private health establishments, all should work together in dispelling the myths, misconceptions, stigma, and discrimination attached to the HIV/AIDS.

With the spread of HIV across the country, more and more positive people are coming to health care centers in the government and as well as in private sectors. It is the responsibility of government to ensure protection to the rights of PLWHAs (People Living with HIV/AIDS), their confidentiality and privacy, and other human rights while providing proper health care and support for these people. If the stigma is eradicated, then the HIV spread can be controlled easily. The right to education and employment of HIV positive people, improved conditions at their workplace will help in decreasing the stigmatization. The government should initiate intensive campaigning and sensitization programmes for doctors, nurses, and paramedical staff to reduce stigmatization. The private hospitals should also rise to the occasion and extend necessary help for the welfare of the positive people. It may take some more years to the general public to accept AIDS victims and to drive out the stigma attached to it.

Ethics of Care and Respect to Positive People:

Ethics of care encompasses providing all medical services to the HIV infected without discrimination. Many dedicated physicians treating HIV cases, take utmost care in treating positive people, with due respect and dignity, and they maintain confidentiality. The discrimination against the HIV infected should come to an end, by employers, landlords, school personnel, and some health care professionals. Thus, centers for Disease Control and Global Programme on AIDS issued guidelines to prevent discrimination and exclusion of HIV infected.[11, 12, 13] and also to prevent spread of HIV at workplace, schools and health care centers. The underlying message of these guidelines is to convince people that HIV could not be casually be transmitted, so there should be no reason for exclusion of infected individuals who are otherwise capable of performing their normal functions.

In the context of health care setting, universal blood and body fluid precautions would protect the health care workers not only from HIV, but also from the far more infectious diseases like Hepatitis B and Hepatitis C, etc., Thus, there was no ground for mandatory foundation for discrimination against persons with HIV. Since the spirit behind this message is not understood by public as well as professionals, the AIDS becomes a center of stigma in every sphere of life. Ethical values and moral principles that rule the people could not even blink at the devil of stigma.

There has been considerable debate on the right to work of the clinicians infected by HIV. This debate has been driven still because of the case of a Florida dentist, who infected his patients. To deny all infected health care workers from clinical work, irrespective of their functions, is irrational and immoral. Many have asserted that physicians whose invasive work can place their patients at some risk ought not to be allowed to engage in these procedures. Are the institutions obligated to screen the health care professionals and if it is so, at what frequency? Is it not necessary to test all health care professionals to safeguard the patients? What about the ethics of informed consent in this situation? [14, 15]

The centers for Disease Control has estimated the risk of transmission from an HIV infected surgeon during an operation between 1 in 42,000.[17] Despite these estimates, there is no documented transmission from an infected health care worker to a patient. The estimates are based on theoretical models. Should the physicians with HIV status disclose it to their patients? Public feels that health professionals should reveal their HIV status to the patients. In one study about 65% of respondents said that they would discontinue all treatment with a health care worker who was HIV infected. Thus, for health care workers disclosure is tantamount to unemployment.[16, 17] One may argue that the health care worker should disclose his status irrespective of loss of job or any other damage that may occur to him. Now it is the turn of the physician to maintain ethical standards of his profession.

Some thinkers raise the question as long as the doctor's HIV positive status does not have the chance of transmission to his patient, what is the wrong if he continuous his practice? One court judgment states: "If there is to be an ultimate arbiter of whether the patient is to be treated invasively by an AIDS positive surgeon, the arbiter will be the fully informed patient".[18]

Other courts have come to different conclusions as to whether as a matter of law a HIV infected physician has a duty to warn patients of his or her condition.[19] Keeping aside the law and judgments every physician is ethically obliged to do justice in the prevailing circumstances.

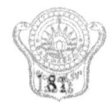

Stigma Remains an Important Problem:

With many other barriers associated with non-adherence of treatment by AIDS patients, stigma remains an important problem in many countries where the resources are limited.

In Soweto[20] and Botswana[21] too stigma is playing an important role in non-adherence. A study in Soweto shows that the odds of obtaining 95% adherence decreased considerably with an increased fear of stigmatization, which involves rejection of the partner or violence against partner. A study in Botswana claimed that in case of 15% patients the stigma interfered with their ability to take medication. Stigma usually posed a barrier for patients who thought they could not take their treatments at home or at work due to fear of detection. Some patients are uncomfortable going to the AIDS clinic for tests and to take drugs because of the confidentiality problem. The same problem is there in India also. People usually expect respect from colleagues, co-workers, neighbors and relatives. They feel that life without respect in the society is a meaningless existence. Hence, they always strive to live with dignity to the extent possible. But AIDS has cruel looks on positive people, and they cannot escape from the tentacles of stigma. Under this back ground, many positive people commit suicide, rather than facing a variety of difficulties and insults from their fellow humans. They avoid going to AIDS clinics, ART centers and popular HIV physicians with a fear of stigma. The change of attitude of the people can only provide solution to this problem, which is silently killing many sensitive and innocent individuals. This is a self-imposed punishment, which is beyond ethics to explain reasons for this tragedy.

In recent times, many cases are coming before the courts concerning claims of negligence. The cases also involve an accusation of a medical practitioner that he did not test the patient for his or her HIV status, or informing the patient's partner about the positive HIV condition and the risk of infection, and the failure to advice against the risk of exposure to accidental infection. The cases are virtually infinite in their variety. When a person has been infected with HIV, it is natural that he or she should look to others to provide financial protection during their lifetime, and protection for their dependants thereafter. Some of the most difficult decisions arise in the area of family law. Cases have been decided whereby access to a child was denied when father was HIV positive[22]. However, the basis of the decision was not due to any great risk to the child. But it is because of the concern of the mother about her child. This was an irrational fear and the judge should not have given effect to it. Court decisions must be based on the real nature of HIV/AIDS. So the prejudice is replaced by knowledge and stereotype, and hence equal justice will prevail in the courts. HIV has brought new points of discussion in law, and demands proper judgment by honourable judges while upholding Justice, which is the need of the hour in the face of AIDS.

Rights of HIV Positive People:

★ Prior consent is needed for HIV testing. But a debate is going on about the methodology to be adopted for universal testing, so as to enhance the efficient preventive measures.

★ The HIV positive status should be kept confidential.

★ As to the discrimination of people with HIV positive status, there is a need for a change in the perception of society towards HIV positive people. It needs continuous awareness projects.

★ To seek legal remedy where the rights of HIV positive people are violated, the voluntary and government organizations are offering free services. But this information is not reaching to all the people who need it at the gross root level.

★ The government should consider sympathetically the issues of HIV positive widows and positive people.

★ Fast Track courts should be provided for the speedy trial of denial of rights and discrimination of the people with HIV/AIDS.

The Role of Society:

★ The society should provide an equal opportunity to positive people and stop discrimination against them.

★ Since HIV/AIDS is a chronic disease, this disease should also be treated like other chronic diseases, such as tuberculosis, diabetes, psoriasis or asthama.

The Role of Media:

The media should play a crucial role in controlling false advertisements about the cure of AIDS and make HIV positive into negative. Deceptive advertisements in the media concerning the cure of AIDS should be stopped. However, the media alone can not stop this practice. The government should have a vigilant watch on such false claims, and suitable legal action should be initiated against such advertisements. The owners of media, both print and electronic should not yield for money and encourage deceptive advertisements, especially on HIV/AIDS. The media persons should feel moral obligation and not to allow fake advertisements for the sake of money. Further, the news agencies should make AIDS awareness programmes as round-the-year activity. [23]

Gender and Stigma:

At one time, AIDS has been considered as an exclusive male disease, but it is now almost equally distributed in both male and females. Though the pandemic is still continuing unabated and infected approximately 38-43 million people by the end of 2009, its pattern is fast changing. [24]

It is identified that over 90% of new infections are now being reported from developing countries; over 75% of adult infections are by heterosexual transmission, and nearly 50% of newer infections in the USA are amongst women. Of these, 84% are in reproductive age group of 15-45 years and only 50% are aware of their infection.

Every 20 seconds a new infection occurs in women somewhere in the world. It is the third leading cause of deaths among women aged 25 to 45 years in the USA, and the most leading cause of deaths among African women in their reproductive age group. The overall AIDS death rate was declined gradually over the years. But, this decrease is at a slower rate among women (17%) than among men (30%). As the HIV epidemic matured in Africa, women started getting infected at higher rate and younger ages in comparison with men. For next few years, it is estimated that HIV epidemic will grow significantly in Southeast Asian countries. The HIV sero prevalence rate among commercial sex workers has been increased from 20% in 1992 to over 60% in 1998 in Mumbai. The sero prevalence of HIV among antenatal clinics has risen to more than 2.5% in Mumbai and is beyond 1% in over 10 states of the country.[25] In India, around 22% of total reported AIDS cases and around 30% of newer HIV infections are among women.

Another issue that has complicated HIV infection among women is pregnancy. In the year 2000, six million pregnant women and 5-10 million children had HIV infections.[26]

The mother to child transmission of virus now accounts for majority of cases of pediatric HIV infection. The issues like rights of pregnant women with regard to mandatory testing, instituting antiretroviral therapy to prevent MTCT (mother to Child Transmission) in the absence of long term antiretroviral therapy for mother, issue of child becomes orphan sooner or later are some of the matters that need a debate to evolve some logical solutions. The problem increases further in countries like India where health systems are over stretched, level of awareness is low, and affordability of antiretroviral therapy is poor. There is gross under recognition of HIV infection in women and actual burden is probably much greater than reported. In many families in India when both husband and wife are HIV positive only husband uses ART, leaving the wife for the nature to take care. When I questioned one woman about the gender inequality, the woman replied that "male life" is more important for taking up the responsibility of family. "Even if I die, what will happen, so why to waste money on me", is the reply of many innocent women, and they are not willing to take treatment for HIV. In the eyes of AIDS ethics, gender equality stands only for statement sake.

AIDS Ambassadors to Fight on Stigma:

Good news from women voice is that the French first lady Carla Bruni Sarkozy, a 40 years old super model turned singer, started to support the Global AIDS campaign with her star power to fight a disease that killed her brother, Virginio in 2006. On the world AIDS day, December 1, 2008, the wife of President Nicholas Sarkozy inaugurated her new mission as the first ambassador to the Geneva based Global fund to fight AIDS, tuberculosis and malaria. In the very early days of epidemic after the death of Hollywood star Rock Hudson, the super star Elizabeth tailor started a massive awareness campaign on AIDS and organized several fundraising programmes to support AIDS victims. This needs further public support. In recent times, in HIV/AIDS homes, some positive women and positive men are being wedded, and it sends a positive message to their people and also to the society around.

Discrimination against HIV positive patients needs some sort of concerted efforts on many fronts to give them space and scope in the mainstream of public life. It is a painful fact that some patients are being discriminated by their own family members. To overcome this menace, many HIV positive people have found a solution on their own and started marriages within their own group.

Schools for HIV Infected Children:

The issue of HIV positive children is now another burning topic in the community. The Chief Minister of Kerala Mr. Oommen Chandy announced that the state Government has decided to start an aided school exclusively for HIV infected children in Thrissur. At the time of inauguration, the school was named as Asha Kiran, a home for HIV positive children. Mr. Chandy said: "the Government would shortly launch the next phase of the anti-AIDS campaign that would focus on rehabilitation of HIV infected people and their families." The programmes of earlier phases were held for creating awareness on HIV and safe sex, he added.

The Chief Minister stressed the role of non-governmental organizations in organizing HIV related campaigns, especially in the rural areas. However, it does not mean that the Government was trying to go back from its responsibilities he said.[27] A similar move must come from the chief ministers of other states in India to solve stigma problem and specially the problems of positive children.

Social Issues, Women and HIV/AIDS:

The link between gender inequalities and women's vulnerability to HIV/AIDS is now a common knowledge. Apart from economic risk factors and biological vulnerability, which put the women at risk for

HIV, there is the complex framework of socio-cultural norms and attitudes, which promote and shape skewed gender relations. These socio-cultural factors put the women at risk by promoting behaviour, which increases the chances of sexual transmission of HIV, and limits the women's ability to engage in HIV preventive behaviours. In several countries, a woman's ignorance of sexual matters is considered a sign of purity. Such an approach restricts women from becoming knowledgeable about their bodies and sexuality, and not able to make choices/decisions regarding their sexual behaviour and consequent reproductive health. Even today, virginity is highly valued, and young couples may engage in unsafe anal sex to prevent pregnancy and safeguard virginity, completely overlooking the risk for HIV. This practice is highly dangerous.

Womanizing becomes a masculine ultimate, which includes multiple partnerships and emphasize male control in sexual relationships. This civilization promotes an increasing risk of HIV in women. In cultures where women are socialized to please men and accept to male authority, may not refuse to engage in unprotective high risk sexual behaviour.

Thus, one could say that the unequal role and status of women predisposes them to the risk of acquiring HIV. However, empowering women by providing them information about sexuality, STDs/HIV/AIDS can help them develop a critical consciousness about their sexuality, which could lead to action to change regressive sexual norms and attitudes that are harmful to them. This needs a constant educational programmes at gross root level, in slums, rural areas and tribal belts where woman are treated like slaves in many families.

Approach to an HIV Positive Patient:

An individual infected with Human Immunodeficiency Virus (HIV) can present to the physician either in asymptomatic phase or more commonly as a symptomatic patient. The asymptomatic person usually comes to know of his/her HIV status during a pre-employment medical check up (usually for overseas jobs), or when offering as a voluntary blood donor, or during antenatal screening. These people require a detailed post test counseling with correct information about HIV infection, the need to change life style, to maintain good health with adequate nutrition and exercise, to avoid infecting others by practicing safe sex, and to have periodic health checkup.

The presentation by symptomatic HIV positives depends on the stage of the HIV illness in which they are first seen.[28] But the asymptomatic stage is more dangerous in spreading HIV to opposite sex or same sex. Silence spread without the knowledge of the carrier brings several ethical issues to forefront. How can we blame the carrier for spreading HIV when he himself does not know about it. But this amounts to torturing the innocent infected.

Human Rights and HIV/AIDS:

AIDS is a global health problem. This modern plague assumes further significance as efforts both in controlling the disease as well as in immuno prophylaxis have not achieved the perfection in results, despite tremendous research both in basic and applied fields.

The raising trend in HIV/AIDS patients in India and their deplorable plight in getting a reasonably satisfactory medical attention should have made the medical fraternity aware of the need to address and uphold human rights while attending on HIV/AIDS patients. In the contemporary society there has been oppression, tyranny and apathy, and indifferent attitude towards AIDS patients, by officials, hospital staff, public health personnel, political leaders, doctors and general public are fueling it further by showing discrimination against HIV/AIDS patients and their family members. When a layman consults his family physician about the HIV infection to his son, many times, the family physicians abruptly make tainted comments without proper understanding on the nature of acquiring HIV infection, which may create prejudice to the father against his son. This sort of irresponsible comments by medical community by their family members and by their colleagues on HIV patients literally echoing a kind of psycho-somatic and psycho-social complex problem, which are very difficult to tackle.

Right to health is one of the fundamental rights of every individual, irrespective of his or her caste, colour, creed, race, and socio-political and economic background. In the recent years we are witnessing an increased life expectancy and appreciable reduction in the threat of infectious diseases because of advanced health care facilities.[29] It is true for AIDS patients also.

However, HIV/AIDS pandemic has created its worst effects due to stigma and discrimination at individual level, family level and community level. Diseases like tuberculosis have re-emerged particularly in a lieu of rampant spread of HIV/AIDS. Lack of interest in the protection of human rights provokes the epidemic because stigma and discrimination further enhanced the impact of epidemic on the people living with HIV/AIDS and their families. [30]

The link between human rights and an individual's health has been pioneered. An individual's right to health demands that the government should provide health care to those who are unable to obtain it on their own. In an effort to prevent unintentional acquiring of HIV infection through infected blood, the Supreme Court of India ordered the establishment of a National Council for blood transfusion.[31]

This council should ensure the licensing of blood banks, and a vigil on professional sale of blood to create an atmosphere of safe blood to the recipient. Now the medical services are included in consumer protection act so as to protect the patient's human rights. Doctors can be held liable for any deficiency of services, in particular, medical negligence. Furthermore, to help and safeguard the rights of an innocent patient, the Human Rights Commission is more vigilant now. In spite of all these measures, HIV positive people are not receiving due attention by the medical community. It is thought that the awareness on human rights helps strengthening the AIDS patients in particular, as it is unlawful to deny emergency services to HIV positive persons. Obviously, any such denial of a person's fundamental right is entitled to compensation.

Of course, who shall listen to the voice of HIV/AIDS patients, who are already under the fear of being discarded from the medicare due to stigma associated with this disease, and the financial constraints? While offering the health services to HIV/AIDS patients some sort of underneath denial often persists. This sort of social discard is unlawful and unwanted. Several disparities among AIDS patients from different backgrounds are also a major problem to tackle. AIDS control organizations provide free anti-retroviral treatment/drugs to AIDS patients belonging only to high HIV prevalent states, whereas clinically similar AIDS patients of low prevalent states are denied the free antiretroviral drugs (ART). This kind of approach, however, discriminates AIDS patients in India belonging to different regions. Therefore, the positive patients should collectively fight for their right of free access to treatment. This issue is recognized by the United Nations General Assembly.[32]

NACO has also included the issue of human rights of HIV/AIDS patients in their policy document, emphasizing the role of states to respect, protect and to fulfill the rights of HIV/AIDS patients. Even without complaint against health providers and health institutions in public and private sector if they found guilty for discriminating against HIV/AIDS, the National and State Human Rights Commissions should act stringently to uphold the justice, because HIV positives are scared to compliant against health providers due to stigma.

The Constitution of India fails to patently grant a fundamental right to privacy but the right has been read into other fundamental rights such as right to life and personal liberty by the Supreme Court. Doctors are expected not to disclose the secrets of the patients that have been learnt during the exercise of professional duty, but these may be disclosed only in the court of law under orders of the presiding judge. Confidentiality between doctor and patient can be breached on two occasions i.e. in the larger interest of community and with the patients' consent. Doctors who have respect to values and who lead a righteous life are in great dilemma when they face such situations. However, in the interest of community, doctors may sometimes cross the boarders of confidentiality. Thus, the HIV status of the persons can be disclosed on any one of the above grounds.

It must be realized that disclosure of HIV positive status would lead to discrimination, and therefore that person is unwilling to take HIV test. Hence, it is of utmost importance to respect the basic rights of people with HIV/AIDS disease. The workers who were discriminated against, and lost their jobs because of their HIV status, can file a suit in a court under pseudonyms.

One argument is that if the prospective bride groom is HIV positive and this fact is known to the doctor, then it is the moral obligation of the doctor to reveal the truth to prospective bride to save her life, though the doctor is supposed to maintain confidentiality.

In India, the fundamental rights of HIV positive patients are at the cross roads because of cultural and religious backgrounds, and attitude of people. Women have increased vulnerability to HIV infection due to pervasive violation of women's rights and dignity, which creates a risk environment for HIV transmission. Thus, empowerment of women is order of the day.[33] A ray of hope is that the empowerment would reduce HIV transmission among women.

It would not be practical without the involvement of men. A solution would be educating the younger generation and other sections of society about human rights. In reality, ignorance, illiteracy, superstitions and several socio-economic factors restrict HIV/AIDS patients to achieve their rights through legal fight. There is an impending need to establish a free legal AIDS service for the HIV/AIDS patients so as to handle complaints from them regarding discrimination and violation of their human rights.

Women in India live in a society which is averse to the very birth of female in the family. The grandmother soon after birth of a child looks with all eagerness the genetalia and in case if she realizes, it is a female child, the grandmother curses the mother and child. One may wonder to note that in some rural areas, the female child will be thrown into dustbin on the road side mercilessly. Many young married women due to AIDS become widows in their teens. Among them, a large percent are thrown out of their in-laws house. Neither are they sparingly welcomed by their own parents. These women may be forced into prostitution or living as an unofficial second spouse to maintain themselves and their children. Hence, economic empowerment to woman helps her for respectable earning, which would create self-confidence and uphold woman's rights.

The positive groups and the associations working for the rights of the HIV positive people should be thoroughly acquainted with all aspects of human rights in relation to AIDS issues.

It is better to educate the public, regarding voluntary testing for HIV so as to save them, and to rescue rest of the community. In this process, if any one is found positive, let us accept them and extend all compassion and love for them without even an iota of stigma and discrimination. Further, assisting them to take proper treatment, minimize social burden of mortality and morbidity. This humanistic approach will be rewarding.

Summary:

AIDS-related stigma or, more simply, AIDS stigma refers to prejudice, discounting, discrediting, and discrimination directed at people perceived to have AIDS or HIV, and the individuals, groups, and communities with which they are associated. AIDS stigma is expressed around the world in a variety of ways, including: ostracism, banishment, rejection and avoidance of people with AIDS (PWAs). The outlines of stigma ranges from discrimination against the PWAs, compulsory HIV tests without prior consent or protection of confidentiality, violence against persons who are supposed to have AIDS or to be infected with HIV to quarantine of persons with HIV. The stigma is not sparing even the AIDS service providers such as clinicians working in the area of HIV/AIDS, laboratory personnel, paramedical staff, nursing staff, the non-governmental organizations working in

AIDS sector and the special AIDS clinics which treat HIV/AIDS patients.

AIDS stigma is effectively universal, but it's form varies from one country to another and one community to another and the specific groups targeted for AIDS stigma vary considerably. Whatever its shape, AIDS stigma inflicts suffering on people and interferes with attempts to fight the AIDS epidemic. Indeed, in the year 1988, Institute of Medicine Panel observed that "the fear of discrimination is a major constraint to the wide acceptance of many potentially effective public health measures in the United States. Same is the case in India. Many AIDS patients do not come to the public and do not attend the counseling clinic or ART clinic due to fear of stigma. People living with the virus are frequently subjected to discrimination and human rights abuses: many have been thrown out of jobs and homes, rejected by family and friends, and some of them have been killed by their village people or by their close relatives. For this reason, in narrating the case studies in this work, all original names of the victims have been changed. In addition to this if one person is found positive in a family the other eligible members in the family are not getting suitable matches to perform marriages due to stigma attached to that family, a highly deplorable condition in several Indian joint families. Children born to positive people are facing a great difficulty to get admissions into the schools and thus it is prohibiting of positive children from studies.

Stigma and discrimination together constitute one of the greatest barriers to deal effectively with the epidemic. They discourage governments from acknowledging or taking timely action against AIDS. They deter individuals from finding out about their HIV status. And they inhibit those who know they are infected from sharing their diagnosis and taking action to protect others and from seeking treatment and care for themselves. Experience in this field teaches us that a strong movement of people living with HIV that affords mutual support and a voice at local, regional and national levels is particularly effective in tackling the stigma and discrimination. Moreover, the presence of treatment makes this task easier too: where there is hope, people are less afraid of AIDS; they are more willing to be tested for HIV, to disclose their status, and to seek care if necessary. We are only at the beginning of this unpredicted challenge to our species. The Asia/Pacific region, which is promised an enormous economic growth in the decades ahead, faces both economic and personal challenges due to AIDS epidemic in the region. Unless behaviour is modified and the spread of HIV is contained what all progress is made until now, may roll back.

References:

1. DC. Jayasuriya, (ed) *"AIDS – Related Legislation in the Context of the Third AIDS Pandemic"*, in "Law, Medicine & Health care", New Delhi, UNDP, 1990) pp. 41-47.

2. Regulations of December 26, 1987 on *"Surveillance and control measures applicable to AIDS"* (Int. Dig. Health. Leg 39, 1988), p 623

3. R. Bayer, and C. Healton "*Controlling AIDS in Cuba: The Logic of Quarantine*", *NEJM*, (320, United States Massachusetts Medical Society. 1989), pp. 1022- 1024.

4. Deccan Chronicle, News paper, December 1, 2008, p. 4

5. The Hindu, News paper, December 1, 2008, p. 4

6. The Hindu, "Bus Fare Concession to Positive People by State Government" July 18, 2010, p.8

7. http://www.gujaratglobal.com/nextSub.php?id=4936&catype=NEWS

8. http://www.expressindia.com/latest-news/govt-hospital-staff-in-up-identify-hivpositive-patient-refuse-aid/464119/

9. http://timesofindia.indiatimes.com/Lucknow/Three_persons_with_AIDS_killed_by_kin/articleshow/3299729.cms

10. http://www.e-pao.net/GP.asp?src=26..070709.jul09

11. Centers for Disease Control recommendations for preventing transmission of infection with human T-lymphotropic virus type III/lymphadenopathy associated virus in workplace. (United States, *MMWR* 1985), 34, pp. 681-686, 691-695.

12. Centers for Disease Control recommendations for preventing transmission of infection with human T-lymphotropic virus type III/lymphadenopathy associated virus during invasive procedures. *MMWR* 1986; 35: P.221-223.

13. N .Daniels, "*HIV infected health care professionals: public threat or public sacrifice*" *Milbank Quarterly* 1992; 3: p. 42.

14. L. Gostin *"HIV infected physicians and the practice of seriously invasive procedures"*. (Hastings Center Report 1989) p: 32-39

15. Estimates of the endemic transmission of hepatitis II virus and HIV to patients by the percutaneous route during invasive surgical and dental procedures, (Atlanta, Georgia, *Centers for Disease Control* 1991).

16. Doctors and AIDS USA, *Newsweek* July 1, 1991, pp 48-52.

17. Gerbert B, Maguire BT, and Hulley SB, (eds), Physicians and AIDS. *JAMA* 1989; 262: 1969-1972.

18. Head KC, Bradley Springer L, and Sklar D *"HIV infected health care worker: Legal, ethical and scientific perspectives"*, (Journal of Emergency Medicine 1995), 2: pp.95-102.

19. Faya V Almaraz 329 Md 435, 620A. 2nd 327; KACV Benson, 1993 "Minn. App. Lexis" 1201.

20. Nachega JB, Stein DM, and Lehman DA, (eds) *"Adherence to antiretroviral therapy in HIV infected adults in Soweto, South Africa"*. (AIDS Res Hum Retroviruses 2004), 20, pp.1053-1056.

21. Weiser SWW, Bangs Berg D, and Thior I (eds), *"Barriers to antiretroviral adherence for patients living with HIV infection and AIDS in Botswana"* (Journal of Acquired Immuno Deficiency Syndrome 2003) 34: pp. 281-288.

22. http://timesofindia.indiatimes.com/news/city/allahabad/Women wage-a-positive-fight/articleshow/4886806.cms

23. In the marriage of B and C (1989) FLC 92, 043 (Family Court of Australia).

24. "UNAIDS Fact sheet" HIV/AIDS. The global Epidemic, December, 2009.

25. Sentinel surveillance data supplied by "National AIDS Control Organization, India 1999."

26. Kotter DP, "*HIV in pregnancy*". "Gastroenterol Clinics of North America" 1998; 27 (1): pp.269-80.

27. The Hindu, News Paper, Dec 2, 2005. p. 3

28. JR Sankaran, "*Approach to an HIV positive patient: Diagnosis and Management of HIV/AIDS:A Clinician's Perspective*" (New Delhi, B.I. Publications, 2005) p-158.

29. Malcolm A, "*HIV related stigma and discrimination - Its form and contents*" Crit Rib Health 8:347-370; 1998.

30. Purohit SD, and Joshi KC: '*HIV/AIDS and human rights; Curr Med Trend*" 8: 1610-1614:2004.

31. Kuman S, Indian Supreme Court demands cleaner blood supply: "Lancet" 347; 114; 1996.

32. "UN General Assembly Special Session Bulletin on HIV/AIDS 2001.

33. Heise L, and Elias C '*Transforming AIDS prevention to meet women's needs - A focus on developing countries.*" "Social Science and Medicine" 40: 1995, 931-943;.

Chapter Seven

Ethical Issues Concerned with AIDS Drugs, Vaccine Trails and Insurance

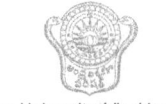

CHAPTER - VII

ETHICAL ISSUES CONCERNED WITH AIDS DRUGS, VACCINE TRAILS AND INSURANCE

Research in pharmacology is an ongoing process to solve several medical problems, to find out new drugs and vaccines, and to discover solutions to improve the quality of human life. In the context of HIV/AIDS, drug trials, vaccine trials, and epidemiological studies do attract a series of scientific, ethical and legal considerations. In any drug trial, usually animals are used first to know the effects and actions of drugs, and once the toxicity of drugs and their adverse affects are completely assessed, subsequently the tests are initiated on humans. To ensure high ethical values in drug trials, ethical committees have been set up. Nevertheless, there has been a stringent criticism on biomedical research. Animal lovers belonging to Blue Cross Organization used to make protests in front of research institutions to stop using animals for research with a view to prevent cruelty towards animals.

It has come to light that some research bodies are recruiting young people under the pretext of giving employment, and using them as guinea pigs for human experimentation.

Is it not unethical to use human beings as experimental subjects without their knowledge and informed consent by paying money to them unlawfully? In situations like AIDS, since the drugs such as ART and HAART by nature are antiretroviral, which reduce the replication of virus, may cause life threatening adverse affects. During the process, the person on experiment may lose sight, may develop cancer, may become psychiatric or may even die abruptly. The moral dilemma involved in the process is, if new drugs are not invented by means of animal and human experimentation, then how the biomedical research would make a progress? On the other hand, how can we justify research on animals and human beings, which may cause a great deal of damage to them?

New forms of treatment usually lead to dramatic self-evident advancement in medicine. Sometimes, instead of doing good to the patients, they may do harm to them. Before they are used with all confidence, their efficacy must be adequately established by clinical trials. Thus, ethical precepts demand that the best available known treatment is to be given to the patients. When no other established competitive treatment is available, then a placebo can be used for the psychological benefit of the patient.

The advance of HIV infection and its ongoing dramatic invasion into the sexually active population of both developed and developing countries has posed many ethical questions and implications of clinical drug trials.

Administration of a Test Vaccine:

When volunteers are being enrolled for HIV vaccine or drug trials, it stigmatizes them in the society. Further, going for a HIV diagnostic test, causes a great deal of psychological stress on the persons concerned. Here the question of confidentiality arises in dealing with HIV test results. Thus, the physician holds the responsibility either to inform or not to inform the test results to the patient. In case he turns to be positive, what would be the implications of the patient, his family and other sexual partners? What would be the social disadvantage to the volunteer who becomes HIV positive not as a result of infection but as a consequence of administration of test vaccine?

Many international agencies, for reasons known to us, prefer to conduct vaccine trials in countries like Africa, India, and Thailand where the volunteers are cheaply available with less expenditure, less legal implications, less responsibility, less post trial follow up, less compensation for possible health damage. It may not apply to every set up, but it looks as though the life of the black volunteers is less valuable or negligible when compared to the life of white people, commented by a journalist. It is a subject of interest, why such research is not guided or controlled by statutory bodies like UNO (United Nations Organization) and FDA (Food and Drug Administration).

In spite of several unethical trials known to the public, there is always pressure on the research community to produce tangible results. While assessing the antiretroviral drug Zidovudine, the initial enthusiasm arose from the results of a single prematurely terminated trial, which indicated that it protected patients from opportunistic infections and death over a period of some 20 weeks.[1]

In India research on HIV/AIDS is guided by the ICMR (Indian Council of Medical Research), following the "Ethical guidelines for biomedical research on human subjects."[2] There are 12 principles laid down under statement on general principles that are common to all areas of biomedical research including HIV/AIDS. They are:

Principle of Essentiality:

This principle states that the intended research on human beings is considered as an absolute necessity, and no other alternative would suffice to carry on the research.

Principle of Information:

The subjects chosen for experimentation should be fully informed about the research and its impact and risks on the subjects.

The subjects used for research retain the right to abstain from further research at anytime irrespective of legal or any other obligations. The principle of informed consent is a cardinal principle and it is to be observed through out the research and the volunteers should be kept informed about the developments in the research.

To make a mature and free choice with an understanding of the consequences of the research, the health care professionals must provide full information about those consequences to the volunteers. Many subjects may refuse to continue in the project if the potential complications are revealed to them.

Since the purpose of information is to enable the subjects or their lawful surrogate to make choices based on an understanding of the consequences, there is an obligation on the part of health care professionals to present the information in such a way that the persons/patients involved in the research are to be properly and fully understand the consequences. The person's mere signing of a consent form saying he or she has been told the facts does not mean informed consent has been obtained. Even though the law accepts such forms as a proof of informed consent, the principles of ethics demand that the health care professional make sure that the patient understands the consequences in terms of the things that are important to him.

Principle of Non-Exploitation:

As a general rule, research subjects are remunerated for their involvement in the research, irrespective of their background and status. Every research should include an inbuilt mechanism for paying compensation to the volunteers through insurance coverage or any other appropriate means to cover every risk foreseeable and unforeseeable. In research, there should be extended treatment, comprehensive after care and appropriate rehabilitative measures. This component of research should be strictly implemented.

Principles of Privacy and Confidentiality:

The identity and the records of human volunteers in a research should be kept confidential to the possible extent, and ensure that they should not suffer from any form of hardship, discrimination or stigmatization as a consequence of participation in a research or experiment. The research body should develop a suitable methodology to maintain privacy and confidentiality.

Principles of Precaution and Risk Minimization:

Utmost care and precaution should be taken at every stage of research experiment to ensure that the research subjects are put to minimal risk and suffering. There should not be any irreversible adverse affects on them for participating in research.

Principle of Professional Competence:

The most competent and qualified persons who are mindful of the ethical considerations in respect of such research and who act with total integrity and impartiality should conduct the research. Selection of the people, who conduct research, is equally crucial.

Principles of Accountability and Transparency:

The research should be conducted in a fair, honest, impartial and transparent manner after full disclosure to those who are associated with the research or experiment. Furthermore, the total records of the research and data collected should be preserved for a reasonable period prescribed, for the purpose of post research monitoring and evaluation or for further research. The records should be available for scrutiny by the appropriate authority if necessary.

Principle of Public Interest:

The research or experiments and their applicative use should be beneficial to entire mankind, but not simply to those who are socially affluent or the research subjects themselves. The application of the results should be uniformly accomplished to all sections of the population.

Principles of Institutional Arrangements:

It should be the duty of all persons connected with the research to ensure that all procedures required are complied with and all institutional arrangements required are made in respect of the research. Further, its application should be in a transparent manner. Also necessary arrangements should be made to preserve the research reports, materials and the relevant data. Research carried out in reputed institutions will add authenticity and sanctity to the work.

Principle of Public Domain:

The results of any research should be brought into the public domain so that the public know about the findings. Public opinion may be invited on sensitive issues and their arguments may be published in the interest of whole population.

Principle of Responsibility:

The professional and moral responsibility should be top on the agenda for any research that is conducted. The outcome of the research or experiment is to be duly monitored and constantly subjected to review if any remedial action is necessary at any stage of the research or its future application that should be properly implemented. This will enhance credentials to the total research.

Principle of Compliance:

Every person engages or associates in conducting research involving the use of human subjects should follow the guidelines specially laid down for such research. To ensure safety and credibility, the persons connected with research or experimentation are supposed to follow the directives and norms prescribed to that area of research and duly complied with.

The violation of these twelve principles raises several questions and doubts about the kind of research that is being done in India or elsewhere, particularly in relation to HIV/AIDS.

Do the research bodies genuinely follow these norms and principles in their research on human persons? Are they meticulously following the guidelines at every stage of the research on HIV/AIDS subjects? Episodes like research on Nigeria Sex workers, reveals that they are used to have sex with HIV positive clients under the pretext that these sex workers have special protection from HIV. Of course, few sex workers might have resistance to HIV infection. How far it is morally justifiable to conduct such a risky research on this deprived class of society? After all, they are also human beings and their life is precious. They also have apprehensions about HIV infections. It is amazing that how the activists, the ethical committees, and scientists who strive for moral values from world over have been dumb in such a sensitive issue and allowed the research.

Similar is the case with the tragic story of Microbicides research on Kenya women in 2007, where by using a product/microbicide supposed to prevent HIV infection, which failed to give intended results. Thus, the innocent women who are used for the research were infected with HIV. The research bodies may say that they would take care of their health, but they cannot take away the trauma, the silent suffering, and the social stigma attached due to HIV positive status. Is it not unethical to conduct such a risky research on feminine gender in particular?

Some researchers may argue that if research is not conducted on human subjects in spite of some risk involved in it, how the science would progress or how the remedial measures would be discovered, or how the future generations would be benefited. It is a big ethical dilemma either to continue the research on human beings or to stop it in the wake of these endangering circumstances.

And also the Zidovudine and Neverapini trials to prevent HIV infection from mother to child transmission may lead to several side effects such as Neverapini resistance among mother group and severe hepatotoxicity.

AIDS Vaccine Trials in India:

In respect of AIDS vaccine trials in India several ethical benchmarks and unanswered questions have emerged. In 2006-07, in phase-I, two preventive AIDS vaccine trails have been launched, the first at the National AIDS Research Institute (NARI) in Pune, and the second in Chennai at the Tuberculosis Research Centre in collaboration with the non-governmental organization YRG-care. In view of the international controversy in Uganda and Thailand trials, these trails in India need to be assessed in terms of the gains made from the standpoint of ethical standards as well as some challenges that need further public discussion.[3]

Some people disagree with the decision of the political establishment and the scientific institutions to provide higher priority to investment in AIDS vaccine trials, but one must acknowledge the achievements in the context of maintaining moral standards in the preparation and conduct of clinical trials. It doesn't matter, even if, such standards were established due to pressure from activists or the international community. The preparatory process for the AIDS vaccine trials was regularly reported in the media. Strategic attempts were made to evolve a "political will" by involving some members of parliament, the Prime Minister's office and the President. Efforts were also made to involve persons with various professional expertise in periodic consultations through an advisory body, some of these contributed actively to laying down the informed consent process. And lastly, at both the trial sites, there was an attempt to ensure greater local involvement through community advisory boards.

The informed consent and participant information documents were drafted using the inputs of diverse stakeholders and experts. It was ensured that all known risks were clearly disclosed and the right to withdraw from the trial at any stage was made very explicit. Several other issues were addressed as well. Thus, guidelines for recruitment were developed to exclude the possibility of coercion and gender imbalance; a recommendation was made to recruit educated persons through public advertisements; a test of comprehension was to be administered; and to avoid the possibility of undue financial incentive, a standard nominal reimbursement of expenses for each visit was fixed for all participants. Participants who became HIV positive during the trial would receive free access to care, support, and treatment, including anti-retroviral therapy, for five years, and an assurance was given that continued access would be advocated for them. The sponsor insured all participants for care, treatment, and compensation for trial related injuries. An independent arbitration board was created to redress trial related complaints, and this includes compensation for injuries and the care of participants who become HIV positive. A stipulation was laid down so that the ethics committee and the arbitration board's recommendations would be respected fully.

Although there is no independent assessment available on the extent to which these standards were actually implemented during the trials, but the fact is that all sponsors agreed to these standards. This system has established a benchmark for all clinical trials taking place in the country. "Research is fundamentally a bunch of failures with an occasional bright light of a success." It is true, but how many lives have to be sacrificed for tiny discoveries?

Some Critical Issues for Discussion:

Before conducting any clinical trial, it is essential to consider whether there is a moral justification for exposing participants to the risks of the trial. Some doubts still persist about the justification for the hasty beginning of the first Phase-I trial at the NARI of the tgAACo9 (code name of the vaccine) a recombinant adeno-associated viral vector based candidate vaccine.

Phase-I trials of the tgAAC09 vaccine had started in December 2003 in Belgium and Germany and their results were awaited in early 2005. Instead of waiting for these results, a trial of the same candidate vaccine, with the same protocol, was started in India on February 7, 2005. On February 22, barely two weeks after the trial was launched in India, targeted Genetics, the company conducting the trials in collaboration with the International AIDS VACCINE Initiative (IAVI) issued a press statement announcing the preliminary results of the Belgium–Germany trials. It states: "The phase-I trial is primarily designed to evaluate safety and tolerability of the vaccine at escalating dose levels. The study is also designed to evaluate immune responses following vaccination. No safety concerns were identified and the vaccine at the doses evaluated was well tolerated. In addition, a single administration of the vaccine at the doses evaluated in this initial study did not elicit significant immune responses."

Since the overseas sponsors of the India trials, IAVI and Targeted Genetics were also involved in the Belgium–Germany trials, it is inconceivable that they did not know of the latter's preliminary findings two weeks before the extension of that trial in India. Did they share this information with the Indian sponsors like the Indian Council of medical Research, the ministry of health and family welfare and the national AIDS control Organization? Did the Indian sponsors ask to examine the data of the Belgium-Germany trials before commencing the trial of the same vaccine in India? This apparent lack of communication raises questions on the nature of the partnership between the Indian and overseas partners.

Under these circumstances, a few months after the trial started, the sponsors in India were compelled to make amendments, including amending the informed consent, which is a gross irregularity. A related question pertains to the complete absence of a "political and scientific will" to systematically develop and test therapeutic vaccines. This is perhaps an inadvertent outcome of depending on a single sponsor. The therapeutic vaccine would pose fewer ethical challenges. The scientific challenges may be comparable, but it would cost less to vaccinate infected persons alone, rather than an entire population. Why is this option kept out of the policy debate?

The field of vaccine development today is driven not entirely by altruistic motives. It is shaped as much by philanthropy as by competitive market interests, global institutional arrangements of intellectual property rights, patents, scientific capabilities and the interests of investors and shareholders. Hence, another critical area that needs public debate is the arrangement between the company holding patents of the candidate vaccines and the government. It is essential that only those candidate vaccines are tried whose technology will be transferred to the host country, with the commodity to be made available at a price that the country can afford. In the absence of specific agreements and mechanisms for accountability even a successful trial may not necessarily benefit the country.

India has become a global hub, or a global laboratory for clinical trials. The reasons are – (i) poverty stricken people for easy money. (ii) most of the volunteers participating in trials are illiterates, and hence medical companies need not provide enough information to the clients especially in AIDS research. Therefore, AIDS activists should drive their attention on these matters in the larger interest of the country. The differences between legal and moral issues have to be considered, especially in an area like AIDS vaccine research.

Most of the new HIV infections are in under-developed and developing countries, and thus AIDS is posing a serious threat not only to the global health but also to the global development. The prevention programmes like health education, condom promotion, clean needle distribution and peer counseling have slowed down the spread of HIV, but these programmes could have not eradicate it. Domestic violence in all countries is to be addressed properly,[4] as this can also contribute for the rapid spread of HIV/AIDS.

Recent advances in treatment have yielded important new AIDS therapies, but the cost and complexity of their use put them out of reach for most people in the countries where they are mostly needed. In a country like India significant access to ART is still a dream.

Nevertheless, free ART centers started throughout the country and 2,82,526 patients are on ART as on 30th November 2009.[2] However, with the improvement in therapy most of the patients are living longer after the diagnosis of AIDS. This has resulted in dramatic decrease in AIDS deaths nationally. For example, in the United States, the AIDS deaths in 1999 were 16,273 as compared to 50,610 deaths in 1995. It remains to be seen whether the decrease in the number of deaths can be sustained over the long term. The availability of quality care and treatment is one key element. In India too the death rate among HIV positives is falling dramatically in comparison with pre HAART era. This state of affairs requires a comprehensive life insurance and health insurance policy so that AIDS patients in developing countries also can have access to the costly combination therapy to lead a long and healthy life.

AIDS: Life Insurance and Ethics:

Between 1980 and 2000, the development and progress in the field of HIV/AIDS is undoubtedly more than 100 fold. Again, from 2000 to 2005 it has further developed to another 100 fold. Enigma behind this disease being behavioral in nature has claimed top seat under communicable diseases of public health importance. There is an increase in the seropositive feature of HIV cases and AIDS cases, which have made a tremendous impact on ethical issues, related to HIV/AIDS.[6] The social stigma attached to AIDS becomes a stumbling block even to take a LIC policy.

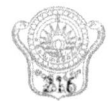

Now HIV/AIDS is about two and half decades old, and it has had a significant effect on almost all the countries of the world. It is threatening to slow down the economic progress of many developing countries. It has wiped out a majority of energetic and young males who are in economically productive age group in many countries of sub-Saharan Africa. Nearly 20 million people have died of AIDS so far and around 45 million are currently living with HIV/AIDS. It is estimated that everyday 15,000 new people are getting HIV infection in the world, and half of them are females, and 90% of these people belong to developing countries. Now the focus is shifting from African to the Asian continent with vast population in India and China showing rising prevalence of HIV. The situation may soon be explosive if adequate measures are not taken. Around 7.2 million people are infected in Asia and of these more than half (3.97 million) are in India.[7] These figures are constantly changing due to the nature of this disease.

The advent of ART has revolutionized the medicare of HIV/AIDS patients. The HAART (Highly Active Anti Retroviral Therapy) has the potential to prolong life, and hence positive people are living near normal life.[8] Thus, there is a great need for health insurance to HIV seropositive individuals. Insurance is a necessity for everyone, but health insurance is very much crucial for HIV positive people not only to obtain medical care but also to pay one's debts after death and to provide relief and support for the dependent spouse and children. Otherwise after the death of the earning member of the family, the principle source of income is lost and several families are thrown into streets.

To lead a healthy life a HIV positive individual, needs nutritious diet, family support, timely laboratory investigations, and regular use of ART with good adherence. For all these components, financial support is of paramount importance. And this aspect can be fulfilled by the life insurance companies, provided they have human face in their approach towards AIDS patients.

It is said that health is wealth. If a person maintains good health, it gives everything to him. In this sense health is an important virtue and one has to purse and maintain it. "Duties of oneself, to preserve one's life, maintain one's health, and develop one's talent, according to Kant, were the most central of obligations."

But unfortunately many insurance companies in India, such as LIC, Bajaj, MetLife and ICICI are not readily accepting insurance to cover HIV positive people under their schemes. Insurance companies like 'STAR' though proactive to give policy to AIDS patients, their area of operations are very limited. Even the popular *'Aarogya Sree'* scheme, introduced by the Government of Andhra Pradesh, is also a form of insurance that has not extended its benefits to AIDS patients. At this point, I would like to question, when many diseases such as renal failure, kidney transplantations, heart attacks, strokes, cancers etc., have been included under insurance benefits, why AIDS disease is set aside? Why it is not included in *'Arogya Sree'* scheme? Such type of discrimination against AIDS people is morally wrong.

This type of discrimination looks as though the life of a person with kidney disease is more precious than the life of an unfortunate AIDS patient. Such disparities and imbalances are not a welcome feature in the health sector. Human life is precious, and if death occurs to a person due to failure of kidney or due to AIDS both are same. If the government equally treats all patients with serious and life threatening, then only AIDS patients would be benefited. At least, government machinery should not treat AIDS disease and AIDS patients as untouchables.

Throughout the World, life and health insurance is essentially a risk allocation contract where the policy holder "transfers certain risks of loss to the insurer, for a monetary consideration[9]." "It is axiomatic that insurance does not cover known losses. Insurance covers the risk of loss.[10]" The industry is usually heavily regulated only by the state[11], unless a particular aspect of insurance is pre-empted by federal law. The same is the case in India.

Insurance is a means of providing protection against financial loss in a great variety of situations. Health insurance helps to pay medical bills. People also can buy insurance to cover unusual types of financial losses. For example, dancers can insure their legs against injury.

Insurance gives the policy holder a sense of security. Many private health insurance companies are coming into market, but not covering HIV positive patients. Usually health insurance pays all or part of the cost of hospitalization, surgery, laboratory tests, medicines and other medical care. However, some diseases are not included for taking policy and health insurance, to which AIDS is joined lately in the list. AIDS is a chronic life long health problem. It involves recurrent expenditures or investigations, anti-retroviral drugs, and treatment for opportunistic infections and so on. As AIDS is not enlisted for claiming insurance benefit, many AIDS victims are facing severe hardships. Though health insurance companies claim that they are in frontline, to rescue in times of need for their policy holders, but these companies are not allowing AIDS patients even to take a policy. This is a deliberate injustice and it amounts to violation of rights of those infected by HIV. Several insurance corporate companies campaign themselves as though they are doing great service to the society. They too have social responsibility. If it is true why they are discriminating the unfortunate positive people? On the one hand the HIV victim can not go to work due to ill health and thereby no earning, and on the other hand, devouring health insurance further subjects him to suffering, lack of proper treatment, starvation and even death. The other pathetic condition is that the life insurance company hesitates to pay the benefit on insured policy by positive patients as per LIC policy guidelines, when they die in an accident or due to related diseases. This is high time for the government to think of an insurance solution to the AIDS patients.

Should an HIV seropositive worker needs to be a bankrupt to be eligible for Medicaid.[12] It looks as if the Medicaid is often the last resort. Medicaid is shallow and inadequate for AIDS patients. Many middle-class Americans are learning the hard way that, in most states, they can qualify only if they are totally disabled and have less than $1,500 in their name. AIDS has shown that we can produce medical miracles for the rich and bare neglect for the poor. AIDS drugs and treatments are priced for rich people and kings, while Medicaid is only for people who have been made paupers.[13] But one thing is true that even Medicaid coverage will not eliminate the problem of (PWAs) people living with AIDS in view of its limitations like, the insurance companies do not pay the medical bills towards vitamins, protein diet, tonics or even health drinks like Horliks, Boost etc., which are very much needed to HIV positive people.

Except in India, in most of the countries of the world, either private companies or governments are offering partial or full insurance coverage schemes. Further, policies against contracting HIV have been developed in case the insured contracts HIV. In Canada, an applicant can pay C$4 and receive a $100,000 policy if the applicant becomes HIV seropositive during a trip. The insured must take two tests – one 14 days after returning from the trip, which should be seronegative; and the other test should be seropositive 180 to 210 days after returning from the tour, and then only the candidate is eligible for claim.

In Italy, an insurance policy has been offered that will cover the applicant if he accidentally gets HIV infection[14], due to positive blood transfusion or accidental needle stick injury. In South Africa, the South African nurses association has initiated short term insurance policies for nurses who may be infected with HIV while on duty. Applicants need not have to take a blood test or a medical check up but need only a signature giving declaration of health.[15]

In Great Britain, critical insurance policy pays a lump sum amount for the persons who suffer from cancer or heart attacks and strokes, but it excludes HIV. Some companies cover HIV if it is contracted through blood transfusion or from a medical occupation.[16]

Within America various insurance companies provide HIV insurance to health care workers who contact HIV in the course of employment. The American medical association offers a nation wide plan of a lump sum insurance amount of up to $500,000 to any physician who contract HIV.[17] In India so far no comprehensive insurance scheme for HIV/AIDS victims has been formulated either by the government owned or private sector insurance companies. It is a large deficiency, which needs appropriate action.

Different types of Insurance Policies:

The Life Partners, Inc., a new business company has formed to deal with "death futures." This is one of the biggest of about 30 companies that invest in policies on their own or match buyers and sellers for fees or (3 to 5 percent) commissions.[18] In this system some companies will purchase life insurance policies of PWA and continue to pay premiums until the death of the insured. So the purchaser becomes the irrevocable beneficiary and the PWA gets remuneration that can be used for treatment or vacation or for any other purpose.

In February 1995, dignity partners, Inc., which had purchased policies from HIV seropositive persons, "closed a $35 million deal" with Ironwood capital partners Ltd.[19] It looks as though that some insurance companies are playing with the lives of people with AIDS. A death can occur too soon or too late. Further, there is a question of how death comes about. There are deaths that are slow and agonizing and deaths that are gentle and graceful.[20] In such cases, it is nothing but gambling with the death of HIV infected persons by insurance companies. How far this business practice is ethically right?

Two young Americans have auctioned their policies in London. The first policy, paying $75,498 is expected to sell for $60,000 and the insured has a life expectancy between 1.5 to 2 years. The second policy worth $100,000 has been auctioned for $90,000, since the insured has only 13 months to live.[21] However, the expectations about the survival of HIV patients may not happen precisely.

Similarly, an HIV seropositive person might obtain more money if he/she auctions it or sell it to a company specialized in purchasing a policy from "people with life threatening conditions."[22]

In a way the life of the positive people is being marketed. In other words, the life of a HIV positive person is kept for sale/auction in the open market for the simple reason that the positive person is in need of money, and he is not sure of his life. This type of unethical business became flourishing, which is based on the sentiments of "life and death". It is a colossal moral dilemma whether to support such actions where the positive persons are under the influence of entering into business deal. At the same time, the companies would like to encash the "situation". It is not only unethical but also brutal to play with the lives of HIV positive people.

In India, for reasons unknown, no insurance company except 'Star' is doing business in a limited way on HIV positive people or People Living With AIDS (PLWAs). It would be a welcoming change if insurance companies come forward and give policies for total care and protection of HIV positive people. We don't know when it will happen or it would be like a day dream.

Insurance Coverage for Negligent Action:

Insurance may cover an HIV seropositive person's negligent actions but not those that are intentional. For example, in the case of homosexuals, Christian Vs. Estate of Rock Hudson,[23] the jury concluded that Hudson's lover should be awarded $21-75 million because Hudson had not informed him of his HIV seropositive status while continuing intimacy.[24]

In some countries, litigation has been viable alternative for HIV seropositive persons with hemophilia. In Netherlands, an individual became HIV seropositive when injected with an unclean needle used to an AIDS patient. The insurer accepted liability and paid $86,000 as compensation and an additional $57,000 for pain and suffering. When the victim rejected the $57,000 and demanded $400,000 the Supreme Court awarded him $170,000 for pain, "the highest amount awarded in the Netherlands."[25] In other countries it is difficult to sue a hospital for negligence concerning HIV seropositive transfusions. The insurance payments will benefit primarily spouses and children of HIV seropositive persons with hemophilia and blood transfusion recipients.

Many innocent women in India have been receiving HIV seropositive transfusions in rural and urban busy hospitals. It is surely because of lack of proper awareness about hasty blood transfusions and the hidden dangers of HIV transmission. The blood banking system in many parts of the country is not efficient due to poor vigilance by the government. In spite of the legislation to check professional blood donation, it is still continuing. In addition to this, owing to greedy nature of the blood bank management, very often it happens, without screening the blood donors for HIV, malaria, hepatitis B, venereal diseases, the blood is being received, sold and transfused. In the era of AIDS accepting unscreened blood is equal to a death sentence. Everyone should condemn this type of immoral business of blood banks.

The hysterectomy (removal of uterus) is a very common operation in many parts of India as a surgical indication for suspicious cases of cancer cervix or uterus or related gynecological health problems. The *Arogya Sree* scheme, the flagship health insurance scheme of the State government of Andhra Pradesh, has funded the removal of over 11,000 uteri through surgical procedure since July 2008 till date all over the State. This is worked out to cover 524 hysterectomies per month. Majority of the hysterectomies were performed upon complaints of white discharge and excessive bleeding by the women, and very few upon discovery of ulcers or wounds in the cervix. Unfortunately this operation is done to many young women in the age group of 25 years by the greedy doctors to earn more money. In this hurry process, operations, accidental HIV seropositive transfusions are happening so often. Because of the social stigma attached to HIV/AIDS, victims of seropositive transfusions are not initiating legal action on hospitals for negligence and positive blood transfusions. The WHO cautioned about the unethical hysterectomies in five districts of Andhra Pradesh — Nalgonda, Karimnagar, Srikakulam, Prakasam, and Kurnool, between December 2008 and February 2009.

It is a sad state of affairs that is going on in the country even after 27 years of HIV history, tests like nucleic acid are not routinely done to identify HIV in the window period. This is another negligent action which can transmit HIV, of course, one in one lakh transfusions. Infecting innocent persons through negligent blood transfusions and negligent sterilization of instruments is a deliberate act of unethical practice by medical professionals. The society should gear up to punish the corresponding culprits before any court or law comes into operation to rescue them.

Of course, insurance companies are doing business to make significant profit on the life of people. One may argue that the insurance companies are helping the people but many times they simply refuse to insure people basing on their background though it's unfair and irrational. Most of the patients who are asymptomatic have many long years ahead of them. Therefore, good number of health insurance companies should come forward to give suitable policies to the seropositive people as they are issuing for many other ailments like heart disease, diabetes mellitus, major operations etc., The basic idea is that the insurance companies should not discriminate the HIV positive people, rather they should extend their reasonable helping hand to them.

HIV/AIDS is one of the most difficult pre-existing health conditions of today, to obtain any type of healthcare prescription or life insurance coverage. In the absence of any social security, people living with HIV/AIDS in India have to face immense difficulties. Medical insurance for infected people in a few districts of the state of Tamilnadu has given them some respite. This experiment needs to be extended to the rest of the country.

India's fight against HIV has reached new milestone with the launching of the first ever medical insurance for people living with HIV (PLHIV). The pilot project initiated by an NGO called Population Services Internationals (PSI) project connect, a programme designed to build public private partnership in combating HIV and tuberculosis in India. The scheme also involves the Karnataka Network of positive people (KNP+) a state level collective of PLHIV and a private insurance company, star health and allied insurance, and it is supported by the United States Agency for International Development (USAID).

The scheme has been opened to a group of 300 PLHIV, with a CD4 count of 300 cells per cubic mm in the six districts of the South Indian state of Karnataka. These are: Bellary, Mangalore, Udupi, Mysore, Bangalore and Kolar. The strength of person's immune system is determined by his/her CD4 count. It tells how far the HIV has advanced, which is also known as T4 count or T-helper cells. Normal CD4 count in adults ranges from 500 to 1500 cells per cubic millimeter of blood. The policy, valid for a year (April 10, 2008 – April 9, 2009) has a premium of Rs.1,511. But PSI has been able to subsidize the premium so that each of the insured has to pay Rs.755.

However, the policy has to be proposed by government agencies, NGOs and other registered bodies working in the area of HIV and the CD4 count should be not less than 300 cells/ cumm.

This pre-requisite is a major problem for many PLHIVs in our country because they cannot come openly declaring themselves as HIV positive to take support of government agencies. Here also, the stigma is a stumbling block for applying and getting relief through health insurance. Thus, the insurance sector has always discriminated against the PLHIVs. The few people who have policies could not disclose their status due to social boycott. Though it is late, than never the government should consider a uniform insurance policy for the PLHIVs with low premium. The HIV blood test should be taken as criteria for giving health policy, rather than the CD4 count which cannot be dependable at all times.

"It is difficult to imagine how the world can grow together and overcome the instabilities and inequalities of global interdependence unless something serious is done to turn the tide on AIDS". As aptly said by the U.S. President, William J Clinton, it is difficult even to convince any insurance company to offer a policy to PLHIVs to continue to have a quality life.

Improving the Quality of Death:

Is there such a thing as an easy or peaceful death?

AIDS has brought many unexplainable sensitive issues into front line. Many times when the test result turns to be HIV positive, young people used to commit suicides. Suicide is a suicide but some people want easy suicide.

"How people die remains in the memory of those who live on" said Dame Cicely Saunders, Founder of the modern hospice movement. Though she earned enormous wealth, her ambition is that everyone should die in a peaceful and painless environment which has not yet been realized. Dying is life's one certainty, yet we often fail to plan for it and go to great lengths to avoid discussing it in a polite company. Is there such a thing as a good death and, if so, do we have the power to arrange it? [26]

In a document entitled "End of life care strategy" brought out by UK department of health, published in July 2008, states that many people do not have a good death, and that there is insufficiency training among health and social care staff to deliver the best care. Suppose a person with AIDS and malignancy would like to have a peaceful death without pain, how it can be possible? And this attracts several ethical dilemmas, particularly in modern medicine.

Hospices provide an excellent model for the end of life, but due to space and funding issues, only 4% of the half a million people are dying in England each year at Hospices, while the majority – 58% die in hospital, and 18% end their lives at home. Seventeen percent die in care homes and 3 percent elsewhere.

"So often we see a moment of surrender in people who are dying. They have accepted that they are not going to win. When people die peacefully they have a beautiful expression on their faces. It gives a sense that they have decided now, to leave this world of pain and hatred, particularly the cancer patients who have suffered so much, it's lovely to know that they are not going to suffer any more. [27]

AIDS patients who wish to end their life prematurely or abruptly, search for several ways as death does not scare them at all. Some of them would like to have touch or gently holding their hand or arm or stroking their forehead by their loved one. Touch is usually one of the last senses to go like hearing. However, death is not seen as a death or sorrowful event in life when people die of HIV. Death in case of AIDS has lost its melancholic nature, and it is treated as a 'boon' and relief to the person. The philosophical explanation and feelings towards death are no more valid in the era of HIV/AIDS. What a pity to HIV/AIDS victims and death and its consequences of these patients.

2009 MDG Report and Future of Insurance Sector:

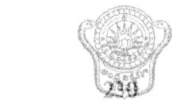

The 2009 MDG (the Millennium Development Goals) report launched in Geneva on 6 July by Secretary-General of UNO Ban Ki-moon warns, despite successes in may areas, the overall progress has been too slow for most of the Millennium Development Goals – the globally agreed targets to halve poverty, hunger, and tackle a host of other social and economic ills to be achieved by 2015.

This year's Millennium Development Goals report delivers a message that should not surprise us but we must take it to heart: "the current economic environment makes achieving the goals even more difficult," Mr. Ban told in the high-level segment of the Economic and Social Council. The Secretary-General called on rich and poor nations to boost efforts to fight poverty and hunger. The 2009 report showed that recent advances are being threatened by the global economic and food crises, which may influence badly the insurance sector. The Secretary-General noted that higher food prices in 2008 have reversed the nearly two-decade trend in reducing hunger. In addition, momentum to reduce overall poverty in the developing world is slowing; tens of millions of people have been pushed into joblessness and greater vulnerability; and some countries stand to miss their poverty reduction goals.

Further, the target for eliminating gender disparities in primary and secondary education by 2005 has already been missed, he noted. Meanwhile, 1.4 billion people must gain access to improved sanitation by 2015 in order to achieve the sanitation target. "We have been moving too slowly to meet our goals," said Mr. Ban. "Yet the report also shows that when we have the right policies, backed by adequate funding and strong political will, actions can yield impressive results." These MDGs have cross section influence due to AIDS burden. AIDS makes people sick, so productivity falls, and it eventually affects the economy of the nation.

HIV/AIDS and Global Economic Crisis:

The well-being of millions of people could be put at risk as HIV prevention and treatment programmes fall victim to funding cutback as a result of the global economic crisis, warns a new report released recently by the UN Programme on HIV/AIDS (UNAIDS) and the World Bank. *The Global Economic Crisis and HIV Prevention and Treatment Programmes: Vulnerabilities and Impact report* says that eight countries – which together are home to more than 60 per cent of all those receiving AIDS treatment – are already facing shortages of antiretroviral drugs or other disruptions to treatment.

In addition, 34 out of the 71 surveyed countries report that HIV prevention programmes focusing on high-risk groups such as sex workers, injecting drug users, and men who have sex with men are already feeling the impact of the crisis. This will continue further. "This is a wake-up call which shows that many of our gains in HIV prevention and treatment could unravel because of the impact of the economic crisis," said Michel Sidibe, UNAIDS Executive Director.

In 2006, the U.N. General Assembly pledged to achieve universal access to comprehensive HIV prevention, treatment, care and support by 2010. According to a news release issued by the agencies, there are no reports of major cuts in donor assistance for 2009. However, it was reported that current funding commitments for treatment programmes in nearly 40 per cent of the countries examined will end in 2009 or

2010. It is feared that external aid will not increase or even be maintained at current levels.

The economic crisis will definitely exert pressure on the life insurance companies to come out with suitable policies for HIV/AIDS infected patients. Obviously the government should come out with innovative schemes to care for HIV/AIDS people on similar lines of *Rajeev-Aarogyasree* as yet AIDS disease is not included in Aarogyasree scheme. Some states in the country offering pensions @ 200/- per month, subsidized food grains and nutritional support to positive people.

Budding Medical and Life Insurance:

Though people living with HIV/AIDS have life insurance in western countries such as USA, positive people in India are denied the right to insure their life. In other words, life insurance companies are totally commercial and are not showing concern for HIV positive persons in India. Drawing attention to the stigma associated with people living with AIDS, many activists asked the government and insurance companies to provide health cover to HIV-positive people.

It is a well known fact that due to the successful use of anti-retroviral therapy (ART), people living with HIV/AIDS are able to live longer while maintaining a higher quality of life. Out of an estimated 2.5 lakh people living in the State of Tamilnadu with AIDS, nearly 40,000 are using ART and it is reaching further to many people. After the opening of the insurance sector to private, nearly 22 companies in India provide life insurance service. It is regrettable, however, that not a single company has come forward to provide insurance coverage for the people living with AIDS. This shows the level of inertia of insurance companies towards HIV/AIDS patients. A debate is continuing among the activists about how insurance coverage is to be offered to the people living with AIDS. These people are not beggars. They want to live with dignity and self-respect. Therefore, they should be provided with life insurance as well as health insurance.

A recent study conducted by AIDS prevention and control project among 667 people living with the disease across 10 districts in Tamil Nadu revealed that they were willing to pay premium for health insurance, but they want subsidized private healthcare instead of government intervention. There is a need to lobby with the government and the insurance sector to ensure life and health insurance to the people living with HIV/AIDS in the country.[25] However, life insurance for HIV/AIDS patients, in the country is still in a preliminary stage only. The USA is now trying to get better health insurance for PLWHAs. If the U.S.President Obama can get universal health care to every body in USA, that would be really a 'wonder'.

The debate on the PLHIV life Insurance is an eye opener for the PLHAs insurability. Life insurance of PLHIV is one of the major social security issues towards the PLHAs rights across the globe. In early 1980s HIV/AIDS is a death sentence. But after the advent of HAART from mid 1990s HIV/AIDS is a manageable chronic disease. Hence these patients need care and support, medication and periodical tests to monitor the disease on a long term basis. To reduce financial burden and mental tension of AIDS patients either in the Government sector or in the private sector, life insurance companies should come forward to give an all-inclusive policy to HIV/AIDS patients to lead a respectable life.

A project "Concern International", with the support of CARE INDIA is implementing a major program towards the PLHIV life insurance in the Salem district of Tamilnadu. Initially the program focused on advocating with the Insurance companies. When no company came forward to design a life insurance project, CARE INDIA and PCI jointly launched "PLHA community mutual," through this program and they are insuring the lives and livelihood of the AIDS people. With the active participation of the Salem district positive network- (SNP+) and other regional level PLHA networks, the "PLHIV community mutual" was strengthened. The community mutual is named as *Jeevodhayam*, a community based micro life insurance product for the PLHIV. This major step was based on the strategic information generated by the PATHWAY program, a major care and support program assisted by Center for Disease Control (CDC).

In this comprehensive pilot program, mortality rate has been reduced with enhanced quality of life among 2334 PLHIV. Early identification, home based care, enhanced health seeking behaviour, and regular OI (Opportunistic Infections) management through mobile clinics, and peer education ensured more than 97% of ART compliance rate, and this programme had positively addressed the survival status of the PLHIV.

Jeevodhyam has two micro insurance models for Rs.5,000 and Rs.10,000 sum assured, with a waiting period of one year in which claims are paid at Rs.2,000 and Rs.3,000. During this period, 172 PLHIVs have positively enrolled, 135 of them on ART and 2 of them on second line drugs. The program experienced four eventualities where the insurance claims of three males and one female PLHIV were settled within twenty four hours through this community based mutual life insurance program.

Jeevodhyam, the community based PLHIV life insurance program is a positive step towards PLHIV insurability. This program, which is in its pilot phase, is expected to be scaled up and similar insurance schemes should come up to cater the day to day needs of PLHIVs[29].

HIV/AIDS and Human Rights:

In view of the discrimination, stigma, and hatred that are being faced by HIV/AIDS patients in their day to day life, apart from life insurance issues, the following internationally protected human rights have been discussed both in the global and local context.

(i) The Right to Life and Survival:

The tragic record of HIV infection and AIDS, links closely to the premature death and denial of a person's right to life. Therefore, the law provides a considerable scope to create and enhance legal claims of AIDS sufferers for prolonged care and treatment, so that they can extend their life.

(ii) The Right to Health Care:

The right to health care is addressed in the economic convention, Article 12(1), which recognizes 'the right of everyone to the enjoyment of the highest attainable standard of physical and mental health.' The Article demonstrates that health care includes the avoidance of HIV infection, and for those who are HIV infected to enjoy rights to have the highest health status. They can also achieve, maintenance of a symptom-free condition, reduction of symptoms in the shortest possible time when they occur, and experience of maximum health following the onset of AIDS. Further, the right to health care includes the best available treatment to postpone mental deterioration associated with AIDS, such as clinical depression and AIDS related dementia. In other words, the conversion of HIV into AIDS may be postponed by maintaining the strong immunity and low infections.

(iii) The right to liberty and security of the person:

In the context of HIV infection, right to liberty and security may appear personal rather than political. However, governmental conduct may directly and indirectly affect the extent to which individuals may maintain their liberty and security against the risk of infection and against inadequate health care services when they are infected. Women's vulnerability to rape in circumstances of military turmoil is well documented[30] Men who intend to rape, whether for political purpose of ethnic dominance or as an act of gender superiority, will not restrain themselves for fear of spreading sexually transmitted diseases, and will not use condoms unless perhaps they fear suffering infection.

In many of the government maintained institutions, such as prisons, mental hospitals and orphanages, the HIV infected suffer discrimination and are denied health care and other services, such as dental and sanitary care. Homosexual rape of prisoners and mental health detainees is a familiar phenomenon. This happens mostly in hostels also. Further, consensual sexual activity is known to take place in single-sex institutions such as prisons and hostels. Institutional authorities frequently refuse to make condoms available, on the ground that such sexual activity is a violation of institutional rules.[31]

But in reality, non availability of condoms increase the risk among these groups. The argument is that supply of condoms amounts to encourage such sexual activities but unprotected sex may augment spread of STIs, HIV infection and HBs Ag.

Drug addiction is also common in many prisons, and because needles are scarce they tend to be shared, aggravating the risk of transmission of HIV infection, hepatitis -B, and hepatitis -C. Prison authorities refuse to implement or permit needle exchange programmes in prisons just as they refuse to allow condom supplies. Such policies violate the rights of victims to security. The authorities fail to recognize sex as a natural part of life and the range of compulsive addictive behaviours. There is a demand from the IV drug users in the prisons, to supply sterilized needles and disposable syringes. But drug use in the prison is against the rules and thus supply of syringes in the prisons would be a day dream of IV drug users.

A common expression of the right to liberty is the right to foreign travel, whether for purposes of business, employment or recreation. An early international reaction to HIV infection and AIDS was to presume that the infection originated outside of their countries,[32] and that they could defend their populations by broader controls on entrants, including requiring evidence that those proposing more than brief visits should be HIV negative. Imposing regulations and refusing to employ the seropositive young persons by some companies, would not only violating the rights of positive people to work, but substantially making them to suffer for want of money that is required for their care, support treatment, and nourishment.

It is not out of place to mention that it is inhuman to disqualify positive people to travel abroad from India for employment. Article 21 of the Constitution of India enjoins that no person shall be deprived of his life or personal liberty except according to procedure established by law. International forums on Human Rights should concentrate on this issue for the welfare of positive people. If it is not redundancy, I would like to disclose about my argument on behalf of the positive people's right to travel abroad for a job or otherwise in the General Assembly of the United Nations Organization in the year 2008.

There is evidence that a significant percentage of foreign travelers are sexually active outside their countries, including businessmen who are incidentally 'entertained'. Compulsory HIV testing may be offensive, and futile when conducted on travelers. Similarly, compulsory testing of immigrants at or after their arrival in a country may violate anti-discrimination principles. Nevertheless, human rights principles do not preclude states from making health clearance a condition for the entry of visitors and immigrants. Barring individuals who present a serious risk of infection to a country's population because of HIV infection may not be different from barring them due to other infections, or on grounds of the costs for their care that may over burden the nationally funded health services. However, this problem involves several sensitive issues like respect for human dignity and sentiments, which needs careful consideration.

(iv) The Right to Freedom from Torture or ill-treatment:

The right to freedom from torture or ill treatment, including freedom from inhuman and degrading treatment, is closely related to liberty and security of the person. It is violation of human rights law, if governments fail to exercise necessary discipline on their military, police, prison, and similar personnel. The inter-American commission on human rights recognized the rape of women by military personnel in Haiti as torture, which would be aggravated when HIV infection is transmitted to victims.[33] Torture tends to be understood as willful cruelty inflicted in direct or indirect pursuit of a public or political purpose. Forcing a lady for sex against her will is a violation of human right.

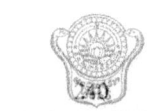

Women face multiple vulnerabilities to sexual and other forms of torture. They are vulnerable to torture in their own right if they defy gender expectations of their subordination and passivity, and become outspoken leaders in protests against political, social and other injustice.

Women's vulnerability to ill treatment in private sector employment can implicate international human rights conventions against ill-treatment, and perhaps indirectly contribute to infection. In many work environments, women become vulnerable to sexual harassment including intercourse which they cannot resist because of their economic dependency on their employers. Beyond sexual abuse, they may be compelled to deal with other activities in unsafe ways that expose them to infection. Further, women who are HIV infected may be compelled to conceal infection and their health vulnerability, and perhaps forego necessary treatment, lest they may forfeit their employment. Enforcement of human rights laws against industrial and related ill treatment would empower such women to preserve their health interest, employment and integrity. Bosses using their employees for sexual needs are not uncommon in many organizations.

(v) The Right to Marry and Found a Family:

The modern international human rights movement was triggered largely by state policies of extermination of ethnic and racial groups, including laws against their intermarriage and on compulsory sterilization. The human rights reaction is the emphasis on rights of marriages and family foundation expressed in all of the leading international, regional and specialized human rights conventions.

Some jurisdictions have reacted to HIV infection by mandating that an HIV test be made a condition of the grant of a license to marry.

Such laws are not only offensive to human rights principles of non-discrimination on grounds of disability, but may be ineffective or dysfunctional if their purpose is to obstruct marriage by infected persons. Of course, this would also offend the right of freedom to marry.

Denial of same-sex marriage may actually be counterproductive, since the spread of HIV infection would be limited by encouraging and facilitating HIV infected partners to remain with each other and not be sexually promiscuous. Marriages among HIV positives in India are a common practice now.

The justification that laws mandating pre-marital HIV testing are designed only to ensure that prospective marriage partners are adequately informed and may be more defensible. The legislation would violate human rights against discrimination against HIV infected persons where it does not apply equally to other sexually transmitted diseases. The duty of states to provide medical treatment, including reproductive technologies, is not established as a positive right by international human rights law. However, where such treatment is provided by a state, the state is bound by the human rights duty not to allow discrimination against people with HIV infection. Human rights principles indicate that women should be permitted to exercise their right to found a family with informed autonomy.

Summary:

In the process of discovery of new drugs and vaccines, experimental studies have to be conducted first on animals and then on human beings. If the drug or vaccine is proved to be toxic on animals then usually studies on human being will be stopped. Animal lovers and organizations such as Blue cross which fights for the rights of the animals, are opposing to conduct research on animals proclaiming that cruelty towards animals is inhuman. How far blue cross would prevent animal experiments is a big question? If animal experiments are not allowed, how the research can make progress in the interest of human welfare?

We often see in the press that human beings are used as experimental subjects even without their knowledge by buying them. It is unethical to use human beings as guinea pigs for experimentation. it is a moral dilemma, how to invent new drugs for the welfare of humanity without conducting drug safety tests on animals or humans. A set of guide lines have been framed by reputed research organizations to follow meticulously but always wide gaps do exist in its implementation.

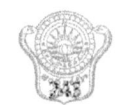

AIDS in the early 1980s is synonymous with death. But with the tremendous discoveries in the therapeutics most of the HIV/AIDS patients are living longer after the diagnosis. In the developed countries, including United States of America, 85% of AIDS patients are leading normal life. In India too the death rate among HIV positives is falling dramatically in comparison with pre-HAART (Highly Active Anti Retroviral Therapy) era. This state of affairs demands a comprehensive life insurance and health insurance policy to the AIDS patients in developing countries also so that they can have access to the costly combination therapy to lead a long and healthy life.

The HIV positive persons, to continue to have a healthy life, need nutritious balanced diet, family support, timely laboratory investigations, and regular use of ART drugs with good adherence. For all these components financial support is of paramount importance. And this aspect can be met by the life insurance and health insurance companies provided they have concern for the welfare of the positive people.

But regrettably almost all insurance companies in India except one or two are not accepting HIV positive people under insurance scheme. The population council, an international organization in association with 'STAR' insurance company with the help of UNDA (United Nations Development Agency) has initiated insurance like scheme for HIV/AIDS patients in a limited way in a limited geographical area in south India.

In the state of Andhra Pradesh "*AROGYA SREE*", is a popular government health scheme. It is also a type of insurance. But it is not covering AIDS patients. At this point, I would like to question, when many diseases such as renal failure, kindly transplantation, heart attacks, strokes, cancers etc., are included in this scheme, why not AIDS disease? It looks as if the life of a person with kidney disease, is more precious than the life of a poor AIDS patient. Different types of insurance coverage have been in practice globally, and such facilities should be extended to all HIV positive needy people in every country to respect the sanctity of human life.

"Death is a death" but what is needed in this context, is to improve the quality of death. Death in case of AIDS patients is not treated as a sorrowful event to their family members and relatives, but it is treated as a 'boon and relief from suffering and stigma'. The UNO and other international institutions struggling to protect human rights and rights of PLWAs, but their efforts have a little blissful impact on the lives of HIV positive people at the practical level.

References:

1. Fischl, M Richarann, D., Grieco, M. et al. The efficacy of azidothymidine ((AZT) in the treatment of patients with AIDS and AIDS related complex: a double blind, placebo – controlled trial. *"New England Journal of Medicine"*, 1987, 317: 185 – 191.

2. *Ethical Guidelines for Biomedical Research Human Subjects"*. Indian Council of Medical Research, 2000, P. 2-8.

3. Amar Jesani, Lester Coutinho Editorial, AIDS vaccine trials in India: ethical bench marks and unanswered questions, *"Ind J Med Ethics"* 2007: 3: 2-3. Amar Jesani, Lester Coutinho Editorial, AIDS vaccine trials in India: ethical bench marks and unanswered questions, *"Ind J Med Ethics"* 2007: 3: 2-3.

4. *"WHO Multi Country Study on Domestic Violence against Women and Women's Health Report"* (Geneva, World Health Organization, 2005)

5. *"NACO NEWS"*, A Newsletter of the National AIDS Control Organization Ministry of Health and Family Welfare Government of India, NeVol. V issue 4 Oct – Dec 2009 page - 2

6. Dr. GN Prabhakara MD, *"Professional Medical Ethics"*, (Hyderabad, Paras Medical Publisher, 2006) P. 193.

7. Usha K. Baveja, *"Diagnosis and Management of HIV/AIDS: A clinician's perspective"*, (New Delhi, B.I. Publications Pvt. Ltd., 2005) P.V.

8. Kutikuppala Surya Rao, Challenges in HIV/AIDS management: systematic review, *"The Antiseptic Estd. 1904, Vol. 103 No.1,"* (Madurai, Professional Publications Pvt. Ltd., 2003), P. 49-54.

9. Ruth E. Kim and Kimball R. McMullin. AIDS and the insurance industry: an evolving resolution of conflicting interests and rights. '7 St. Louis U. Pub. L. Rev.' 155, 155(1988).

10. Sapp. V. Paul Revere Life Ins. Co., 1994 *"U.S. App. LEXIS 15219(9th cir)."* The court granted the insurance company Summary judgment when an HIV seropositive person had not disclosed his pre-existing HIV seropositive status even though he had not been asked about HIV on the life insurance applications.

11. The Mc Carran-Ferguson Regulation Act, 15 U.S.C 1011-1015, et. seq. (1988).

12. Lisa M. Tonery, "AIDS: a crisis in health care financing." 40 Fed'N Ins. and Corp. Couns. Q. 1990; 133:146, 1990. Approximately 40 per cent of all individuals with HIV receive health coverage

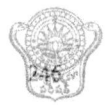

through Medicaid, a federal entitlement programme paid for by the federal, State and local governments.

13. Henry A. Waxman. Introduction to symposium on AIDS. 49 Ohio State "Law Journal" 1989; 877-878. HIV seropositive people are eight times more likely to have lost health insurance than HIV negative people. Michael T. Isbell. Health Care Reform Lessons from the HIV Epidemic. Lambda Legal Defense and Education Fund, 1993:69.

14. Italy: Reale Mutua provides cover against risk of contracting AIDS, "Italia Oggi" 1995 March 31.

15. Cas St. Leger. Questions over AIDS insurance plan for SA nurses, "Sunday Times" 1994 Sep. P. 11-15.

16. Helen Pridham. As state pay-outs shrink, more people are insuring their health critically important. "The Herald" (Glasgow) 1995 Aug. P. 12-20.

17. AMA offers HIV insurance for U.S. doctors, "Reuter Lib. Rpt" 1992, P.12.

18. Leslie Scism and Jeffrey Taylor: SFC questions insurance deals for the dying, "Wall Street Journal" 1994, Aug. 18:B1.

19. Cecile Gutscher, New Class of Investment cashes in on Terminally Ill, "Ariz. Republic" 1995 Apr. 23:E7.

20. Samuel Gorovitz, Dealing with Dying: Doctors' dilemmas, "Moral Conflict and Medical care", Oxford University Press, 1982, P. 153.

21. Jon Ashworth. AIDS victims put life policies up for sale, Sunday Times 1994 Aug. 6. Prudential Insurance of America will pay

about 95 per cent of a policy's face value for an insured that has less than six months to live. Greg Steinmez. New Companies are forming to buy policies of AIDS patients, "*Wall Street Journal*" 1992 Jul. 31:4.

22. "*Insurance Leaflet*", supra n81:10.

23. Y.V.Satyanarayana, "*Ethics: Theory and Practice*", (Delhi, Pearson, 2010), p.183.

24. "*Christian V. Sheft*", (Cal. Super. Ct. Feb. 17.1989)

25. Jury award is sharply cut in Hudson AIDS suit, "New York Times" 1989 Apr. 22:7. Hudson's lover settled for an undisclosed amount while the appeals were pending. Press Association News file 1993, Apr.1

26. "*Insurance Research Literature*" 1993, Aug.1

27. N. Ram ed, "*The Hindu*" June 10 (Chennai, The Hindu group, 2009) (agreement with Guardian Newspapers Limited, 2009). P.9

28. N. Ram ed, "*The Hindu*" June 10, (Chennai, The Hindu group, 2009) (Guardian Newspapers Limited, 2009). P. 10

29. http://"*timesofindia.indiatimes.com*"/Chennai/People-with-HIV-need-life-cover-say-experts/articleshow/4710981.cms

30. S.Ramkumar,e-mail:pciramkumar@gmail.com. Program Manager – PATHWAY TN/AP.http://health.groups.yahoo.com / group / "*AIDS – INDIA*" / message / 10437

31. Swiss s, Griller JE. Rape as a crime of war; a medical perspective: "*JAME*". 1993; 270:612-615.

32. Allyn and Bacon, *"Meier RF crime and society"* (Boston: 1989) P. 414-5

33. Correctional services Canada, HIV/AIDS in prisons *"Final Report of the expert Committee on AIDS AND PRISONS"*, (Ottawa: Minister of supply and services Canada, 1994).

@@@@@

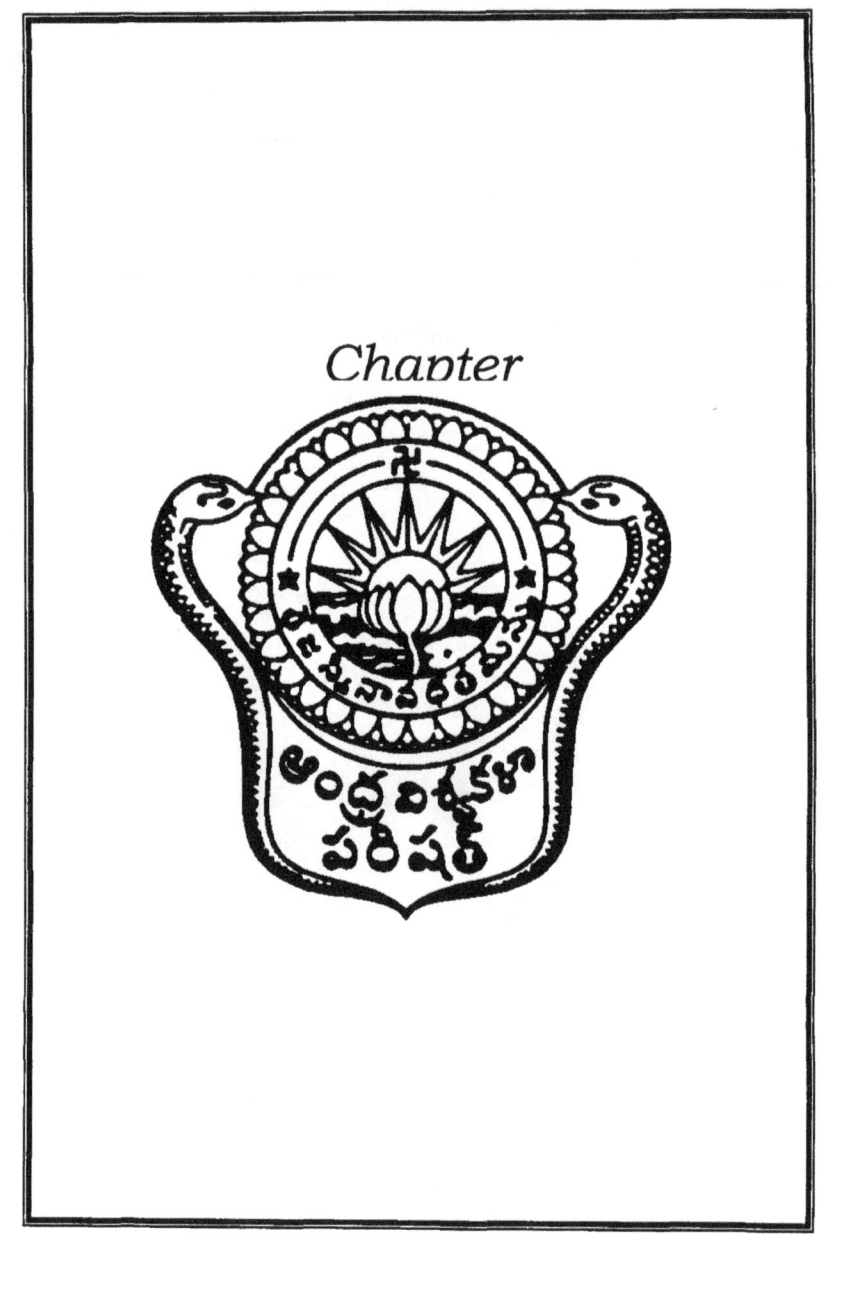

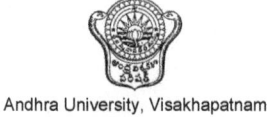

Chapter

CHAPTER - VIII

CONCLUSION

At different periods of history, humanity has been witnessed several forms of epidemics such as leprosy, plague, small pox, and in recent times HIV/AIDS, which is threatening the survival of humans.

Leprosy was a highly stigmatizing disease for centuries due to its horrifying nature of physical disfigurement, and no cure was available to it until the twentieth century. Millions of people across continents became victims to the terrible epidemic of plague. Small pox, which is one of the most devastating diseases known to humanity swept across continents, decimating populations and changing the course of history. However, the World Health Assembly, in 1988 declared that the world is free from such a horrifying disease.

In the contemporary times, HIV/AIDS, another frightening and deadly disease, struck the world in 1981. No disease in human history has created so much of horror, ambiguity, suspicion, and several ethical issues than the HIV/AIDS. It is an on going battle between human genius and HIV virus. Until and unless man conquers HIV virus and discovers pertinent solutions for this pandemic, the life becomes miserable for millions of HIV victims throughout the world.

Gandhi brought freedom to India through his method of Satyagraha or non-violent non-cooperation. But the people of present generation of India need one more freedom, that is, freedom from the clutches of AIDS. In this context, Gandhi's philosophy of Satyagraha movement has to be directed towards "Break the silence." It is the 'silence' that fuels the spread of HIV/AIDS. It is the 'silence' on sexual relationships that promotes the transmission of HIV. It is the 'silence' against the use of 'condom' that is the culprit for high incidence of HIV among adolescents engaging in 'casual sex'. Therefore, breaking the silence creates right awareness to conquer HIV/AIDS.

The impact created by AIDS in all spheres of human life, caused a global turbulence to the very fundamental right of humans, that is, the right to live respectfully. The ethical challenges that are being encountered by AIDS infected, AIDS affected, and AIDS surrounded are innumerable. Children Affected by AIDS (CABA) do face numerous problems in their day to day life. They need special solutions to overcome those problems. Every person must work hard and dedicate himself or herself to create a "world free of AIDS" in every dimension.

It is said: "Those who fail to read history are destined to suffer the repetition of its mistakes." From the times immemorial, man has been struggling to control diseases. Henry Siegerist, one of the medical historians, stated: 'every culture has developed a system of medicine, and medical history is but one aspect of the history of culture.'[1] Dubos goes one step further and says: 'ancient medicine was the mother of sciences and played a large role in the integration of early cultures.'[2]

Since there is an organic relationship between medicine and human advancement, any account of medicine at a given period should be viewed in contrast to the civilization and human advancement of that time i.e. philosophy, religion, economic conditions, form of education, science, and aspirations of the people.

Thus, the Medicial Scince from antiquity has developed leaps and bounds till today with a number of discoveries to improve the quality of life of the modern man. In this process, many ethical issues that are contrary to human value system have been emerging at every stage of development.

On the one hand man is conquered the very secrets of creation by mapping the double helical structure of DNA, on the other hand several viruses, such as HIV, SAARS, and H1N1 (Swine flu) are declaring ferocious war on human beings and threatening the very survival of man with a greater speed than man's expeditions. Therefore, there is a need to discuss the ethical values and principles and examine how they are useful in framing certain rules and procedures of medical profession in general and dealing the AIDS patients in particular.

Dr. Haldon Mahler, the then head of the WHO, three decades ago aptly said: "We are running scared …. (I can) not imagine a worse health problem in this century. We stand nakedly in front of a very serious pandemic as mortal as any pandemic as there ever has been. I don't know any greater killer than AIDS, not to speak of its psychological, social, and economic maiming." AIDS is continuing its supremacy over the human intelligence till today. Though AIDS was identified in 1981, more wide spread public and medical attention developed some what later. By mid 1990s a serious exploration of questions about the threat to public health, and the ethics of private and public policy responses surfaced for debate. Also complex issues like the ethics and human experimentation, non compliance in AIDS research, hiding the fact of HIV positivism and getting married to maintain their prestige in society, the fate of children born with HIV, and some other problems related to AIDS are the greatest challenges of contemporary human society.

The early views about AIDS were based on substantially wrong information, and misconceptions against persons with AIDS, and the solutions they found are most inhuman. The solutions such as--- banishment to an island, tattooing of carriers, quarantine and wholesale exclusion, dismissal from work places and so on. Even now there is no change or improvement over the past views, rather they are intensified. For example, Australia is not permitting positive people for entry into their country. One can imagine how that society was nervous and shivered to the AIDS epidemic.

Proposals such as mandatory screening of every person for HIV, to close gay bath houses, to criminalize certain sexual activities that transmit AIDS, to tattoo positive people, to banish the HIV carriers – all these steps are nothing but the coercive restrictions on the liberty of many innocent persons, based on suspicion that those persons may carry the virus. In the process, axe is always hanging on the neck of innocents in the form of AIDS. Unfortunately, more awareness or unwanted publicity is created on the misconceptions and rumors on HIV/AIDS, rather than the real facts or scientific information of AIDS.

Scientists have achieved fantastic breakthrough in the fields of molecular biology and genetics. There have been significant advances in anti-microbial therapy but medical men are still haunted by the fear of infectious diseases. Many infections like small pox and guinea worm have been totally eradicated, and polio and leprosy are on the verge of eradication/elimination. But, we still get new infections and re-emerge of certain old forgotten infections from time to time.

Now, HIV/AIDS is more than two decades old, and has had significant effect on every country in the world, and it is threatening to slow down the economic progress. It has wiped out a majority of male population of economically productive age groups in many countries of sub-Saharan Africa.

Sir William Osler, once coined a dictum that "Physician who knew syphilis in all its manifestations knew the entire medicine". It means that the physician who is familiar with the diagnosis and available treatment for the wide range of clinical manifestations of infection with T-pallidum, syphilis was at the frontiers of biomedical sciences. The same is true of HIV/AIDS today. Late Dr.Jonathan M. Mann (Director, Global Programme for AIDS) once said: "Knowing AIDS is to know medicine." Knowing AIDS in all its manifestations is a complex, creative, and continuously evolving process. A clinician caring for people living with HIV/AIDS must be aware of at least three elements: 'realities of the disease, the diagnostic and therapeutic capacity of modern scientific medicine, and the psychological and social dimensions of the disease.'

Contrary to this, many physicians are not updating their knowledge, particularly, in the area of HIV/AIDS. When an HIV positive patient consults them, they discourage the patient and his family members or relatives with outdated statements such as, "there are no medicines for AIDS" or "there is no treatment for AIDS" and "whatever you spend on AIDS patient is a waste", "AIDS patients die within few years" and so on. Some family doctors without applying their mind and learning the latest developments in AIDS management are terrifying the AIDS infected and affected with their half knowledge. They are carried away by some notions or baseless rumors such as "by touching AIDS patients AIDS can be transmitted" or by talking to AIDS patients or by sharing the bathrooms of AIDS patients, AIDS can be transmitted and so on. Regrettably some of the so called physicians of Allopathy, Ayurveda, Homeopathy, Unani and alternative medicines are propagating such superstitions and suspecting messages. Honestly speaking, this sort of unscientific propaganda on HIV/AIDS has been victimizing the HIV infected and affected, and it's the stumbling block for the affective prevention and control of AIDS, and it is the prime reason for increasing stigma.

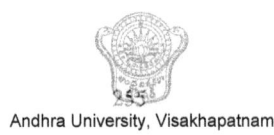

The governments and many international bodies have been organizing awareness camps for the general public, but it is the right time that the health care personnel of all the systems of medicine should be sensitized periodically with the new inventions in the area of AIDS so that the stigma problem can be tackled effectively.

Should a doctor with insufficient knowledge have a right to comment on AIDS patients? Is it not immoral and against the spirit of Hypocritic oath to demoralize and discourage the HIV patients? In recent times, instead of extending their services to HIV positive patients, many doctors are refusing to attend on them and leaving them to their fate. This kind of behaviour may be due to their own inhibitions and false fears about HIV/AIDS, and many surgeons, orthopedicians, obstetricians and gynecologists are not even touching the positive patient, and leave them alone without conducting surgeries. This trend needs radical change, and the doctors should respect the right to life and dignity of HIV positive people.

Recently, several cases are being filed in the human rights court against doctors for negligence and abstaining from treating positive patients. The impact of HIV/AIDS on families, communities, doctors and nations has been well documented.

Paternalism and Autonomy of the Patient:

The conflict between respect for autonomy of the patient and the physician's desire to help patient by controlling his freedom causes the problem of paternalism. The word paternalism is derived from the Latin word *"pater"* means "father". In its dictionary meaning, it refers to a ruling or controlling of others in a way that a father controls his children.

In the context of health care ethics, paternalism involves acting without consent, or overriding a person's wishes, in order to benefit the patient or at least to prevent harm to the patient. Thus, there are two elements involved in paternalism:-

1) The absence of consent of the patient.
2) The beneficent motive of the physician to the welfare of his patient.

From an ethical point of view, the proponents of individual autonomy reject the right of health care providers to apply paternalism, because health care professionals certainly do not have the right to enforce value judgments on the patient on the ground that "doctor knows the best to his patients".

The doctor-patient relationship is quite different from the relationship between parent and child. Active intervention of one person into the affairs of another, without respect for one's right to choose oneself autonomously is unreasonable and unjustifiable.

The doctrine of informed consent is simple and clear on the surface. If the patient understands what the physician proposes to do, and the patient gives his consent to its being done, then the medical intervention is not imposed on the patient, in violation of his autonomy. This procedure of gaining informed consent not only shows physician's consideration to respect the patient's autonomy, but also protects the physician against the charge of imposing treatment on the patient who did not want to take that treatment. In other words, it protects the physician against the charge of assault.

In order to gain a clear idea of what is informed consent, we have to make a distinction between the two parts – informing and consenting. Informing is the duty of the physician and consenting is the duty of the patient.

Recent empirical studies have shown that the cognitive capacities of patients are often diminished by the circumstances of their illness and hospitalization. It is the general complaint of the patients that they have been told nothing about their illness or the surgery that they have faced, yet the medical records show that they have been provided with detailed information and a good understanding of the medical circumstances.

J.S. Mill, the utilitarian philosopher, strongly opposes paternalism and says: "no one else is likely to know better than a given individual what is best for that individual to choose." Mill believes that there is a positive value in the exercise of autonomous choice, so it is better for a person to make a choice in his own behalf than for someone else to impose his choice on him. Immanuel Kant says that human beings are 'autonomous' beings, and they have the ability to decide what is right and what must be done, and therefore, they must be left alone to take their own decisions. Many thinkers believe that paternalistic intervention in another person's affairs, except under very special circumstances, is violation of the other person's rights.

Some thinkers who reject this position argue that it is allowable to intervene in another person's life so long as that intervention serves the interests of the other person. They say that doing good is more important and such intervention is justified. But the price one must pay for holding such a position is precisely a diminished level of respect for liberty and independence that constitutes the very foundation on which autonomy rests. Respect for persons, for their liberty, and their right to express a freely chosen course of action, supports the principle of autonomy.

The argument that patient's knowledge is always imperfect, and imperfect knowledge is inadequate to allow patients to make rational decision about their treatment may not stand valid. Most patients have enough understanding of the medical aspects of their circumstances to exercise reasonable choice. Moreover, the spectrum of understanding is likely depends on the quality of the physician's efforts to induce understanding in the patient. The better the physician is an educator of the patient, the stronger the case for respecting the autonomy of the patient.

The argument that the goal of the patient and the health care professionals is the same, that is, to maximize the health of the patient, and therefore, the choice made by the physician is the best one, is an erroneous argument. The argument that a physician and a patient share common objective do not nullify the patient's right to freedom of choice or autonomous decision.

The argument that some patients can be harmed by the provision of information about their conditions, I think, has substantial force to be considered. In some cases, the patient may be weekend, both physically and psychologically by his health condition, and he is in the care of the physician whose primary responsibility is to protect and advance the interests of his patient. Under such conditions, it is reasonable or even obligatory to withhold the truth from the patient, on the ground that the risk of harm is as great as to override the demands of honesty and patient's autonomy.

Code of Ethics for Medical Practice in Relation to HIV/AIDS:

The HIV/AIDS epidemic is not merely a health issue but also a challenge that influences the social, political, economic, cultural, ethical, and legal parameters of the society. Many medical practitioners are reluctant to accept HIV positive individuals when they come for consultation. Medical practice should not discriminate the patients on the basis of the disease from which they are suffering. But HIV / AIDS has brought a clear apathy towards positive people. This attitude of the current medical profession has been led to many unethical practices by non-qualified as well as qualified doctors. Therefore, it is necessary to practice highest possible ethical standards, both in Medical practice and in medical research to prevent another disaster relating to HIV/AIDS.[3] The HIV Testing and confidentiality about its results is utmost important to avoid troubles related to social stigma. Physicians and Infectious Diseases consultants have to formulate infection control policies and ethical guidelines to protect the medical professionals as well as the patients. HIV-Infected Patients should be treated with due respect by the Physicians and nursing staff. The regulatory Processes and structures in the States and the Central Government have to be designed suitably. There should be a disciplinary body to take action against those people who violate the ethical guidelines both in private as well as public medical institutions. This needs constant vigil and watch in the interest of the medical profession and the public. If necessary, we have to import success stories from elsewhere in the world and strictly implement ethical values in medical profession in general, and in HIV/AIDS related issues in particular.

Ethical Issues in Relation to AIDS Orphans:

In a community, when the AIDS patients' die, their children miss the emotional support of their parents, and the burden of taking care of the children falls on other family members, and all these things become a vicious circle of unpleasant events.

According to UNICEF estimates, about 15 million children below the age of 18 years have lost one or both parents due to HIV/AIDS. The children, who lost their parents, not only lose the warmth, love and affection but also deprived of the concern and care of their parents and family security. In addition to the physical, emotional and psychological trauma, the children become victims of hunger, no access to education or health care, not be able to meet their basic needs, and they may likely be subjected to physical, social and emotional abuse, including physical violence and land grabbing.[4] In the worst cases they may be subjected to sexual abuses.

When parents become sick or die due to HIV/AIDS, the inherited stigma and sickness may further hurt these children for no fault of theirs. The society is so cruel that it haunts these innocent children till their last breath who are HIV infected or affected. The people who have service motive, the civil societies, and the governments should think humanly about the plight of these orphans and come forward for the rescue of the HIV positive children. Many ethical problems are being confronted to rehabilitate the children or to give them for adoption. Eligible parents are also not coming forward to adopt such children. Their entire childhood is inhumanly thrown into desert.

HIV/AIDS Children and their Burden on Grandparents:

In many African and Asian countries, including India, the death of either parent or both parents left their children on the mercy of grandmother or grandfather. In countries like Zambia and Zimbabwe, grandfather and grandson have to lead a solitary life in a hut because there are no other young individuals exist in any hamlet. Added to this, the grandfather has no energy, no income, and the grandson is equally feeble and both are interdependent. Hundreds of villages were totally wiped out as most of the young persons died, and millions of hectors of agricultural land has been deserted with no crops as there is no one to cultivate those lands. AIDS has been creating a ghastly landscape of collapsed families; broken human relations; devastated economies and demoralized societies. Some critics may not accept it, but it is the ground reality and 'the time' alone can witness the victory of man over the deadly AIDS.

A child for no fault of his/her is taking birth on this earth as positive child, because of the mistake committed by his/her parents. A positive child has to lead a life of innumerable health problems due to compromised immunity, and also face the cruel stigma and discrimination of the society. Life becomes a lonely long battle for him, if the diseased parents of the child die prematurely.

Is it not morally wrong on the part of the parents to give birth to a positive child? A positive child will be a curse to the public, and also a burden to the community. Whatever projects and rehabilitation measures are being implemented for the welfare of the positive children, the blow on their physical, mental, social, and psychological growth is beyond repair by any body.

HIV/AIDS and the Role of Media:

By the mid-1990s, or more than a decade after the earliest HIV cases were reported, HIV/AIDS had become just another health story for media, but one view is that media often amplify the issues while reporting on this pandemic. Therefore, the media should be trained property in the use of sensitive language on HIV and AIDS.

FM radio is now popularly being used to address many issues on HIV like depression among women and providing them access to special counseling. The Radio announcer sends messages through popular songs to tackle key issues on HIV/AIDS, and counselors are available on hand to discuss the disease on-air.

There are still many people especially in rural areas who have little or no knowledge about HIV/AIDS. The media should focus on educating rural people on the facts about HIV/AIDS.

Global economic crisis is touching every aspect of human life. Funding to fight AIDS, to create awareness on AIDS, to conduct research on HIV and to discover potent AIDS vaccine is drastically cut down. If media is properly conscious about its role it can bring miracles in the attitude of people with its positive stories. To dispel stigma, both print and electronic media should play responsible role. Media and ethics is the current hot topic of discussion at every platform. Hence, media in the area of HIV/AIDS is the mirror of whole human nature.

Guidelines for Media Coverage:

While increasing media coverage on issues related to HIV/AIDS has supported advocacy in this area, there are many examples of inaccurate and unethical reporting. Newspapers and the audiovisual media have often published easily identifiable pictures of people affected by HIV, including children without their consent. Inaccurate reporting has contributed to stigma experienced by people with HIV or affected by it.

On November 16, 2008, the press Council of India released a set of guidelines for the media to report on HIV/AIDS. These guidelines received a mixed response from the activists and journalists.

The document of Press Council of India highlights the need for accuracy in reporting on this complex and often technical subject. It also presents a framework for reporting. It says that the positive stories should be highlighted, and stereotype reporting should be avoided. The reporters should not focus on how individuals acquired the virus, and erroneous language such as 'dreadful disease' and 'AIDS carrier' must not be used. It is essential to respect confidentiality and the privacy of patients and family members who are interviewed, and their consent must be taken when using photographs, names and stories. The miracle cure reports should be avoided by the press.

The guidelines suggest the media 'to show people living with HIV in a positive manner by portraying them as individuals rather than victims, without giving their identity or photos.

It is absolutely necessary to take consent before publishing the faces. However, there are circumstances in which positive people choose to come into public as the positive community needs to be visible to inspire others. Panos, an international media network, is dedicated to promote quality reporting on HIV/AIDS. Mr.Loon Gangte, one of the members of the Delhi network of positive people, and his family members have given consent to publish their photographs and their story in a book, brought out by Panos. Their intention was that their life may throw light on more people to protect themselves from HIV.

Other guidelines for media coverage of HIV/AIDS focus on helping journalists to improve their skills rather than listing "do's and don'ts". The International Federation of Journalists has been working sincerely for training the journalists, providing them access to correct source of information, and creating conditions for good journalism.[5]

Psychological Support and Counseling:

People diagnosed with HIV infection or AIDS and their family members are confronted by a host of problems that call for emotional and practical support. Anxiety about the spread of infection, physical isolation, hospitalization, discrimination within the community or family, loss of housing, interruption of education, financial problems, the physical effects of illness, disease progression, loss of relationships, bereavement, anger, loneliness, and depression are the problems of these people, which need proper solution. These problems may be intermittent, both for the persons with HIV/AIDS and for those providing care for them. In fact, those problems are not always predictable which produce physical and emotional stress. In such a condition counseling to these people serves two main functions — the first one being the provision of social and psychological support, and the second thing is the prevention of HIV infection and its transmission to other people. Counseling is also particularly helpful in identifying the circumstances under which these problems are likely to be present, and in helping the person to deal with those issues in a proactive fashion. Further, counseling can help the person to react gently to these problems as and when they arise. It is important to remember that counseling incorporates a process of empowerment for the persons with HIV. In spite of living with HIV infection, a proper counseling would help the positive people to lead a productive and independent life.

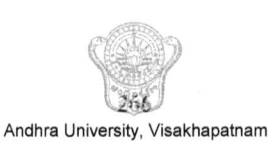

Where people cannot see beyond their HIV infection, counseling can assist them to normalize aspects of their lives that they may otherwise overlook. Counseling should help those affected by HIV to live fully and productively, by enabling them to resume (or assume) authority over their own lives and decision making. Problems can often be placed in a new light, which needs a more creative approach to find solutions and decision making. Counselors may often find themselves in the role of "patient advocate", generating a therapeutic strength in individuals, families or communities by their support. Enabling people to remain active in their work, in their education, in their families and friends, facilitate to reduce dependence on health and social services and reduce the psychological problems.[6]

Rational Suicide:

Some patients with HIV disease want to discuss the option of rational suicide with their primary caregivers and treating HIV physicians. According to one survey conducted on HIV infected patients, 67% of the respondents indicated that they had considered rational suicide as option for themselves. Among these respondents, suicide feelings and depression were not necessarily related. Rational suicide and euthanasia are extremely controversial issues within the frame-work of medical profession.

Nonetheless, medical practitioners must realize the sufferings of many HIV positive patients, and they may consider suicide as an option for them at some point of time in their life. Thus, it is an important issue for the medical practitioners to examine the feelings of AIDS patients, because they are likely to express their feelings to the doctors. Though the law does not permit for assisted rational suicide or euthanasia, it is a matter to be debated seriously at all levels. For a human being, the quality of life is more important than merely staying alive, when life becomes miserable, painful, and worthless.[7]

Home Based Care and Moral Issues:

In the context of care of HIV positives, I would like to discuss about a successful home based care, that is, the Tanzanian model. The home based care (HBC) team consists of a nurse from the local clinic, a voluntary community worker, and a driver and they are accompanied by a supervising nurse from the main clinic. This Tanzanian tem during their first home visit, entered a darkened room where they saw a woman, who was severely dehydrated and not able to move. When the nurse tried to give some water to the woman, she showed the medicines given to her, but she was unable to take them as she has no water or food.

They visited the second house where there was a mother and her daughter. The mother had recently started on ARVs but when they went into the house, she looked so tired and drained. She did not take her ARV that morning knowing that she must eat some food before taking the drugs. But there was no food in the house and also no money to buy. The nurse brought few bags of porridge meal, which the women's 12 year old daughter began to prepare, who was her only support. Before the mother started on the ARV treatment, she was very weak to attend to any work, or to take care of her daughter and herself.

Hence, her daughter stopped going to the school. As the ARV gave her dramatic relief, she could come back to her work and her daughter could return to school. Yet, the grinding poverty in which they are forced to live, threatened the efficacy of the treatment.

Finally, they visited to check on the recovery of John, a young boy, who had been fighting a serious HIV infection. Both his parents died because of AIDS, and his own HIV positive status had made him vulnerable to a series of infections and illnesses. Although he had shown great resilience in recovering from them over a period, at the age of 12 years, he looks like the size of an average 7 or 8 years boy. He questions the HBC team whether they would make him well enough to return to school? His only hope was to receive early ARV. Although the clinic is equipped with moderate resources to place limited number of children on ARVs, the number of children who needed the treatment far outnumbered the resources available, and the clinic was forced to choose whom to treat and whom to leave to die. John is living with an uncle and his family is in a desperately poor condition to meet two meals a day. How to put John on ARV drugs, without enough food in the house to eat, is a big question? ARV without sufficient food will be a failure.

By looking into these three episodes, we can imagine the deplorable conditions of the HIV infected children in Dares Salam, of Tanzania.[8] On the one hand they are suffering from HIV, on the other they have no food or parents to extend their love. This type of scene may be replicated in India very soon as the epidemic has a shift from

Africa to Asia. Is it not unethical on the part of HIV parents to beget children and subject them to numerous hardships and sufferings? Such irresponsible behaviour of the parents opens several social and ethical issues. When the HIV positive orphan children are increasing in number, they will be a burden to the society. Their sickness and untimely death will eventually result in the dearth of human resources of the country. When there are no children, there would be no adolescence, and without youth no country can progress. We cannot imagine a world with a large number of sick children and insufficient number of youth, and such a world society would be a sick society, which prevents the progress of human civilization.

Prostitution – HIV/AIDS – Ethical Issues:

Prostitution is as old as human civilization with different names at different times. According to available statistics it is estimated that in India there are about three to five million prostitutes in the flesh trade. On an average four to ten clients are being entertained in a day,[8] and some clients do not like to use condom. When they are insisted to wear a condom, it is learnt that some guys question: how does a person enjoy a chocolate with its wrapper? Thus, one such positive client is enough to infect several prostitutes and thereby a number of her customers.

It is a fact that the HIV virus is virtually killing thousands of men and women involved in prostitution. Most of the prostitutes are forcefully dragged into it for a variety of reasons, but the most important factor is poverty. It is observed that several women are forced into prostitution because of desertion by their husbands or lovers. Faced with the crude realities of life, these women might be in search of some alternative means of earning for sustenance. Many parents are keen to perform their daughter's marriage at a very tender age and send them to in-law's house. As a result of child marriages, many young married women became widows in their teens, and some of them are thrown out of their in-laws houses' and as a last resort, these young women will land in prostitution to maintain themselves and their children.

The other side of the story is that in a considerable number of instances the husbands are forcing their wives to prostitution for their selfish and unethical gains. At the time of Hindu marriage, the bridegroom while tying the sacred thread *"tali* or *mangalasutra"* on the neck of bride, at the witness of *Panchabhutas* (Earth, Sky, Air, Water, and Fire) and takes oath *"Dharmecha, Ardhecha, Kamecha, Mokshecha ...Nathi charami, nathi charam, nathi charami,"* which means, O lady, by accepting me as your husband, you will live with me till death. Hence to endow you with wifehood, I am holding your hand. The four deities Bhag, Aryama, Savita and Pusha have handed you over to me to carry out all the household duties (*Gruhasthashram*). But, such sacred words and holy promise made in the midst of huge gathering of people, comprising of relatives, friends and unseen Gods, will be buried into ashes, by the husband when he sends or sells his wife for flesh trade. What a great injustice has been done to such women? How unethical practice it is? When a lady came into the bosom of a husband, all the way leaving behind, her birth place, parents, brothers and sisters, relatives, childhood friends, memorable environment like hills, crop fields, springs, and rivers, and if the husband is dumping her into prostitution violating all moral values and norms of a family bondage, what a malicious and immoral behaviour it is? The society as well as the law should appropriately punish such men.

According to Kant, it is morally objectionable to sell or use another person's body to attain some selfish benefit. He says, 'we should never use human beings as mere property or simply as instruments. We must always recognize and respect humanity in others. Humans should not be used as a means to an end.' If someone sells a woman to a brothel house, then there is a possibility for that woman to be infected by some sort of virus, including HIV.

There are women belonging to some communities, whose traditional occupation is prostitution. *Kalavatulu, a community* in Andhra Pradesh, is known for spicy flesh trade. In some communities the eldest daughter is forced into prostitution at an early age to support the family. Some of the young poor girls while taking into jobs in marketing sector are also being sexually exploited by the employers. Many such women turn into 'call girls' serving the clients who come to stay in five star hotels. They mostly lead an unmarried life once for all.

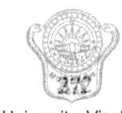

In metro cities many college girls are also known to be working as 'escorts' for tourists and indulge in prostitution, and lead a very lavish and luxurious life. It has been found that several girls from professional colleges who stay far away from their homes also take up this profession for earning more money.

Organized sex trade is well known in India. Many young girls when they come to cities in search of jobs are recruited into this profession without their choice and consent. The girl child born to a prostitute is welcomed by her mother, the brothel-keeper, and the pimps as she would be a potential source of future income. The child prostitution starts around puberty. The estimated eight million children of the prostitution trade have no other option than to follow the profession of their mothers as an occupation. Given the present situation of HIV/AIDS in the country, many of these child prostitutes are being HIV infected either from their infected mothers or through their customers who engage them for sex at a very tender age.

The *devadasi* system is still prevalent in large scale, particularly among the economically and socially weaker sections of the society in Andhra Pradesh, Orissa, Tamilnadu, and in some other states. Young girls are offered to the temples at the age of nine or ten without their consent. These girls are being sexually exploited even before they reach puberty by the so called elders of the village or by some priests of the temples. It is a prestige symbol to have first night with such girls. The village chief or the landlord will purchase the first sex with a girl after her first menstruation by giving prize money. There is also a blind belief that by having intercourse with a virgin the sexually transmitted diseases and AIDS will be completely cured. This misconception is the driving force behind many child rapes in India. Whether it is a call girl, *devadasi* or *kalavati* by whatever name one may call, most of these girls used to move from one city to other city, one hotel to other hotel and one brothel house to other brothel house as new faces are a great attraction to the clients and they get more money. In this process, HIV/AIDS spreads like a wild fire in the community. Some husbands who stay in cities without their wives for months together on employment may go to a sex worker for recreation and acquire infection, and when they go back to their native place on a vacation, they are infecting their innocent wives. It is rampant among construction workers and skilled workers, who leave their family in the village and come to the cities for search of job, where they earn more money and indulge in prostitution. Living lonely far away from wife on a job, and indulging in extramarital sex, and spoiling their wives' health with deadly diseases is absolutely an unethical practice.

Homosexuals, Lesbians and Ethical Perspectives:

Instead of vaginal sex that what nature orders all other sexual perversions are unethical and immoral. This is the viewpoint of almost all the religions. Therefore, the sexual practices among homosexuals and lesbians by and large are against the natural order. But they argue that it is their fundamental right to engage in sexual activity of their own choice. The other argument is that as long as it is a consensual sex between two adults, there is no sin to have sex between two persons of the same sex. Nevertheless, AIDS has brought into surface these activities of darkness. Spread of HIV among homosexuals and lesbians is a big concern today. In fact, the very first four cases of AIDS reported in the world were from homosexuals, and at that time it was called as 'gay disease'.

Several cases of HIV infection through homosexual and lesbian activities have been reported by study teams conducting researches in various pars of India. The population of gays and lesbians runs into thousands in India. They have their own groups and associations. They also publish periodicals which are being distributed. In fact, in the year 1994, a national seminar of homosexuals in the country, the first of its kind was held in Mumbai.

Eunuchs:

Eunuchs have a unique history of working in the kingdoms of Nawabs (Muslim kings). Eunuchs have been widely engaged for sexual gratifications, particularly by gay men and lesbians. Eunuchs also run brothel houses and provide sexual entertainments in five star hotels and holiday resorts. It is estimated that there are about 1.8 million eunuchs in India, most of them are castrated men or school and college going boys. Estimates show that about 40,000 castrations take place in India every year, and out of these people three-fourths die of infection caused due to the crude practice, which has undertaken by eunuchs themselves, or by a barber. Eunuchs also form part of the potential high risk group for the transmission of HIV virus, because they involve in sexual activities with men and women, adolescent street children, and drug addicts. Mostly they engage in anal intercourse and oral sex.

Child Prostitution in Visakhapatnam (India):

Even though there is an Act that protects children from prostitution in India, the Immoral Traffic Prevention Act of 1987, there are many children who are still living as prostitutes. In India, sexual exploitation of children has its roots in traditional practices, beliefs, and gender discrimination. (Jubilee Action)

There are many causes for child prostitution in India out of which three main reasons were identified.

1. Girls were dedicated to the village goddess by their parents at a very young age, and these girls are servants of God known as (Devdasis), since they are married to the God. After the girl is married to a God she may not marry any human being and turns as prostitute.
2. Extreme poverty makes the parents, husband, or siblings to sell the girl in exchange of an insignificant amount of money.
3. Child marriages are common even today in some communities, and in the name of the marriage parents sell their girls for prostitution.

"Child prostitution is the ultimate denial of the rights of the child," said by Dr. Jon E Rhode, UNICEF representative in India. In this background, the author and Stefania Forner a researcher, Pharmacy/Clinical Analysis at Federal University of Santa Catarina, Florianopolis, Brazil, studied about child prostitution in Visakhapatnam during March -- August 2006. Out of 150 street children surveyed who are moving around railway station, bus complex, and parks in the old town area, and Ramakrishna Beach, 6 girls (4%) in the age group of 11-14 years and 9 boys (6%) in the age group of 10-15 years were found engaged in child prostitution. If a similar study is done in other metropolitan cities the quantum of the problem of child prostitution will come to light.

Adolescent street children, and drug addicts in India, are at a greater risk of getting infected with the HIV virus because of their alleged involvement in sexual activities among themselves or by visiting prostitutes. It is estimated that about 50 percent of HIV infection in the country is projected to be occurring in the age group of 10 to 24 years. Several studies conducted on school children, street children, young drug addicts, and alcohol addicts across the country revealed that they indulge in sexual activities at tender ages. Engaging children for sexual activity, who are at tender age, innocent, and pure, is highly immoral and such an activity must be curbed by the government.

HIV in Prisons:

Throughout the world, homosexual activity is being reported in the prisons. Indian Prisons are no exception for this. Several countries have initiated action for the free supply of condoms, and Israel has gone to the extent of considering a proposal to allow heterosexual activities in the prisons by permitting the spouses of Prisoners to visit them once in a week. It is unfortunate that our policy makers and authorities do not want to bring changes in the existing sexual practices among prisoners in all the jails. Since August 20, 2010 on an experimental basis the jail authorities of Anantapur (India), an open jail, started permitting spouses of prisoners to have family life in jails on particular days. It is welcome move to bring psychological harmony among prisoners. According to the press release of the project director of Andhra Pradesh AIDS Control Society report, dated March 23, 2010, out of three hundred thousand prisoners (three lakhs) existing in the Andhra Pradesh prisons, 267 HIV cases found positive, and 1195 prisoners are suffering from different sexually transmitted diseases. Spreading HIV/AIDS and STDs in prisons is causing great worry. The ART is being supplied by the government for 22 prisoners in Charlapalli, 27 prisoners in Warangal, 16 prisoners in Rajahmundry, 34 prisoners in Visakhapatnam and 20 prisoners in Sangareddy[10]. Supplying of condoms to prisoners is a controversial issue. However, Andhra Pradesh Government AIDS control project has been supplying free condoms to the prisoners with a good intention to prevent spread of HIV/AIDS and STI (Sexually Transmitted Infections), but not with the intention of encouraging sexual activity in the prisons.

Persons employed in armed forces – military, air force, navy, and paramilitary forces, have been indulging in homosexual, heterosexual, and bisexual activities not only in foreign countries but also in India. Since these sections are mostly away from their spouses and the desire for sex is to be satisfied these practices are universal. We have a considerable number of documented positive cases among these people.

Sex Education in Schools:

The WHO suggests that school health education programmes should contain lessons on sexual health, reproductive health, and

HIV/AIDS and STD, taking into account the cultural and educational values of the society. But unfortunately many states in India are not interested to introduce sex education in schools. In many places parent associations bitterly opposed this proposal. They argue that sex education to adolescents may provoke the hidden instinct in them, which may ultimately corrupt the young minds. But many countries like Australia have implemented sex education endorsed by the Roman Catholic Church.

The Indian Scriptures – Foundation of Ethics:

The ancient Hindu scriptures emphasize the art of living by following the ethical principles and moral values. The Vedas, the Upanishads, the Mahabharata, and the Gita, proclaimed the ethics oriented family life. The ancient Hindu ethical thinkers designed, purusarthas or cardinal values, to maintain a balance between the physical, psychic, and spiritual aspects of human life. If every Indian practices these principles and values, and order their lives in accordance with the value system of our society, the present generation of people could overcome most of the social evils that are threatening human survival.

Excessive desire for sexual pleasure and perversions of sex seems to be in total opposition to the order of the nature. No religion teaches abuse of sex, but people disregard the principles of moral order, and paving the way for the spread of HIV/AIDS.

Marriage, as an institution, is a device for the adoration and expression of love for one another. According to Hinduism, true love between a man and a woman is the union of soul and body and it lasts as long as life lost. S.Radhakrishnan says: "The unity between a man and woman is not merely a physical unity, but a unity of both mind and heart. It is the law of love that binds them together... We cannot live entirely to ourselves. Apart from the biological side, we need a life-partner with whom we can communicate and exchange our deepest ideas, share our inner most thoughts and feelings, and share intellectual sorrows and pleasures."[9]

The union between a man and a woman is not an end in itself, but it is the means of gaining self-fulfillment of both... They have to live together intimately and affectionately all through their life. One must develop the culture to understand the other, and if necessary, to sacrifice one for the other.[10]

According to J.S.Mill, the British utilitarian philosopher, an ideal marriage mirrors the ideal relationship between a husband and wife; they must show toleration for each other's tastes and habits and be well-behaved with one another.[11] As long as wife and husband are mutually faithful to each other, there is no place for HIV/AIDS through heterosexual route.

ABC Theory to Drive Away HIV/AIDS:

'A' stands for "abstinence" of sexual relations before marriage. This message is the foundation for upholding and practicing of moral values. Contrary to this message, several research studies conducted specially on college students, revealed the fact that 24% boys and 18% girls had premarital sex in India in several metropolitan cities such as Mumbai, Delhi, Bangalore, and Hyderabad.

When the Supreme Court of India gave favourable judgment on March 24, 2010 saying that "no illegality is involved in live-in relationship between majors", or "sex before marriage," once again several controversies raised in our country. A much-publicized statement of south Indian film actress Khusboo on premarital sex, virginity, and live-in relationships came for some positive interpretation from the Supreme Court, which said that there was nothing illegal in live-in relationships between adults. Many orthodox Indians and religious organizations disapproved this verdict saying that the Indian family system and the sacredness of the institution of marriage will be collapsed with this judgment.

'B' stands for "be faithful." After marriage the wife and husband should be mutually faithful to each other. Faithfulness to one another is the very foundation of marriage system. Extramarital sex in India is contributing up to 9 to 11 percent of HIV transmission. This is a crack for the trusted mammoth building of family fabric in India.

'C' stands for 'condom' use. When the partners fail to follow the theory of 'A' abstinence of sex before marriage, and theory of 'B' 'Be faithful' after marriage, the 'use of condom' is advised to prevent the deadly HIV/AIDS. Advising the use of condom is deemed to be unethical, because it promotes prostitution, and provides fuel for multiple sexual partnerships. In this context, a moral conflict arises between promoting the use of condom to save the life of a person, and discouraging the use of condom to preserve the value system of the family or 'divine bliss of sexual relationship' In such a situation, the utilitarian thinkers held that saving the life of a person outweighs the value system of the family or divine order.

The young boys and girls, who are very emotionally attached to one another, are not bothering for the value of life, and involve in a haphazard sex. It has also come to light that the young adolescents do trust each other deeply, and thus they do not bother to use condoms. The youth used to argue that the use of condoms breaks the intimacy and the mutual trust between the lovers. This type of attitude is one of the reasons for the prevalence of HIV/AIDS upto 81% in the age group of 15-24 years.

In a vast country like India, which is known for its rich cultural and high standards of values and family system, AIDS is posing a big challenge to the physicians, parents, social activities, policy makers, political leaders, religious heads, academicians, and researchers to control the spread of deadly virus. In view of its nature, the routes of transmission, and the everlasting stigma attached to it, all those people involved in AIDS treatment and control are also equally facing many problems. It is regrettable to say that for a momentary pleasure of sexual intercourse, we forget everything and bringing death sentence on us. Our knowledge, our ethical values, and our wisdom could not prevent us indulging in immoral sexual acts, which ultimately lead us to feel guilty, worries, tensions, stigma, shame, and silent suffering. In the process of momentary sexual pleasure, some may be infected or killed with a disease like HIV/AIDS. Basically, what is needed today in India is to accept the fact that we practice double standards in our value system. The so called rich culture, heritage, family values, religious principals betray the poor, illiterate, and ignorant Indians. Therefore, to rebuild the Indian value system, we should change our attitude, and try to protect the value based family structure, to save the lives of millions of people from the clutches of AIDS.

In India any strategy to prevent HIV/AIDS, should be based on the fact that Indian people are second to none in their sexual life style. Whether one accepts the fact or not, there are several sexual perversions, lesbians, homosexuals, sex workers who are minors, and many reported cases of incest in our society. The modern India is no more a virgin land, to some extent, if not completely.

It is high time for every Indian, irrespective of his or her political background, or religious affiliations, should realize the importance of the ethical values taught by our ancient ethical thinkers and practice them to get rid of HIV/AIDS, and to safeguard the health of our present and the future generation of people.

In early 1980's, a mystifying disease shocked the first bunch of homosexuals but it didn't generate either big bang sound, or volcano voice, or earthquake noise, or Tsunami ultrasonic sound, but it is a direct blow on the humanity as a whole. In the medical terminology that disease is named as AIDS (Acquired Immuno Deficiency Syndrome) by scientists. But, as a student of philosophy, I would consider and elaborate it giving a different meaning to each letter of AIDS:A-aggressive, I–inhuman, D–destructive, S–sorrowful. Thus, AIDS is an aggressive, inhuman, destructive, and sorrowful disease. This disease rapped human dignity and freedom of the victims. For a religious person, it looks as the curse of the God.

AIDS patients are surrounded by fear, hatred, animosity and dislike. People are scared to see the HIV positives from a distance as if the wind blowing over them may infect others. Many people did not know about the anatomy, the physiology, or the science of HIV. But unfortunately the same is the case with some medical personnel till today. Intentionally, these few medical men fuel the entire society and in turn contaminate each and every one they encounter, with their half and erratic knowledge on AIDS.

Patients generally expect the utmost care and concern, and dedicated service from their doctors all the time, day and night. But doctor is also a human being, and he may not satisfy his patients by attending round the clock, without loosing temper.

A young widow came to my clinic recently and told me that she got married to a young man two months ago who was HIV negative. Immediately I asked her "did you tell him about your positive status"? She said 'no.' Then, I asked her why you did not inform him before marriage? "Had I told him, he might not have married me" was her reply. She further said with coolness: "if he continues to be negative he may suspect and during the course of time he leaves me. If he also turns to be a positive, then there will not be any blame on me from his side. As the AIDS drugs are available now, if he becomes positive then we both can use medicines." What a crude and cruel woman she is? Instead of wishing welfare and good health to her husband, she wishes that her husband should get HIV infection from her. Her argument is that she should not be blamed or insulted by her husband for her HIV status. What ethical values and family responsibilities will nurture between such couples, where the life partner have such a cruel and selfish idea in her mind. The lady looks so innocent, but the deep rooted feelings in her heart and mind are venomous and ill-intentional. To infect a person with HIV virus intentionally is not only brutal but also highly unethical.

In some other instance a woman, who is also a widow came to me with an appeal that "Please see that I survive at least till my daughter's marriage is performed, otherwise she becomes a destitute. She has no father who died of AIDS and if I die she becomes an orphan. Therefore, I am prepared to spend even Rs.10,000/- PM towards my medicines. Doctor please "save me". She is not rich, and therefore, I recommended her to an ART centre where she can get free medicines. She bluntly refused my suggestion stating that if she goes to a public government hospital her identity may be reveled, and her daughter may not get a good alliance. She questioned me, who will give a bridegroom to the daughter of a positive mother? That is her concern for her daughter. She is a small vender, who sells biscuits, chocolates, etc. on a pushcart in one of the rehabilitation colonies of steel plant.

Criminalization and AIDS:

At least 600 HIV-positive people have been convicted for transmitting HIV or exposing others to it, according to figures presented to a satellite session of the AIDS 2010 conference on July 19, 2010 in Vienna.

The figures are based on the data gathered by GNP+ (the Global Network of People Living with HIV), which has been running a Global Criminalization Scan to monitor prosecutions since 2005. It has recorded prosecutions in 50 countries, with those in North America and Western Europe leading the way. However, that there is a growing trend in African countries to criminalize transmission of the virus. In total, 45 countries have laws that specifically criminalize HIV transmission or exposure.

Susan Timberlake of UNAIDS told the session that it was now a "corporate priority" of the organization to "remove punitive laws, policies, practices, stigma and discrimination that block effective responses to HIV".[12]

The Problems Created by AIDS and Appropriate Solutions:

The problems connected to HIV/AIDS are of many types. They are as follows:

1. Individual level 2. Family oriented 3. Society based 4. Health related 5.Financial centered 6.Psychological issues 7.Immoral conduct 8.Discrimination 9.Anguish 10.Melancholy 11.Despair and 12.Suicide.

As a practicing physician and as a specialist in the treatment of HIV/AIDS, I would suggest the following Ten Commandments to prevent HIV/AIDS:

1. Adultery Indiscriminate Dearest Sex (A.I.D.S) is to be avoided.
2. Although the premarital sex is legitimated by Supreme Court of India, sex before marriage should be avoided.
3. A Man and a woman, who are living together without marriage temporarily or on a contract, both must be cautious as HIV is lurking in casual sex.
4. Extramarital sex and multiple sex partners should be avoided.
5. Every person should be faithful to the life partner. In other words, mutual faith and trust between couples should be honestly maintained.
6. When partners fail to be faithful and random sex is inevitable one should always use condoms to avoid the risk of HIV and other infections.
7. All narcotic drug injections, intramuscular, intravenous or subcutaneous should be avoided to the extent possible.
8. Each and every blood transfusion should be organized only after implementing scrupulously the WHO guidelines, such as testing for HIV before accepting the blood from the donor.
9. As a whole safe sex, safe needle, safe blood, safe motherhood, safe shaving will prevent HIV/AIDS.
10. The prospective bride and bridegroom should undergo HIV testing before marriage for the good of both.

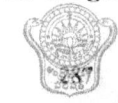

The Need to show Human Concern in the Treatment of HIV/AIDS:

Physicians, health care personnel, nurses, and family members should develop and show concern, love, kindness, care and, amicability towards positive people, which will boost their morale and contribute to the longevity of life.

In this context, I propose, a bunch of duties to be followed by the physicians, or health care persons who are attending on HIV/AIDS patients. Physicians should be kind and cool towards the patients. It means the physician should maintain patience when he is listening to their feelings, sufferings, and opinion. The physician should respect the patients, must be truthful, and transparent in his investigations and treatment. Health care professionals should be pleasant, pure hearted, and punctual in solving the day to day problems of the patients. Doctors must be passionate, and profoundly share sorrows and joys of the patients to the extent possible. Physician must be answerable for all procedures proposed or done for the betterment of patients. The physician attending on the patients should always be available to the patients, and abide by the principles of medical ethics in upholding the self-respect and human dignity of HIV positive persons.

HIV/AIDS is opening the Pandora box of human nature and human relations. The sufferings of the HIV positive people due to stigma and discrimination are indescribable. To sum up, the social stigma attached to AIDS kills more people than the AIDS disease itself.

Medical Practice and Decline of Ethical Values:

The use of expensive laboratory tests, in preference to clinical examination for diagnosis, became a common practice today. The failure to understand the natural history of the patient's illness is resulting in hasty investigations and thoughtless therapy. The use of expensive tests may also be gaining prominence because of the 'incentives' offered by laboratories and scan centers to the doctors. A portion of the fees paid by the patient to the centre is passed on to the clinician. This unethical practice is camouflaged by the use of terms such as 'fees for clinical assessment' or 'provision of clinical details'. Several specialist doctors working in government hospitals rush to the private nursing homes during their office hours to treat patients, rather than taking care of their patients in the teaching hospitals. It became a common practice in several cities, since the corporate hospitals are offering 'fat fees' to the consultants.

If people with power and wealth become the goal of the average physician, then the poor will not find a proper place in the minds and hearts of the physicians. At present, the medical tourism is flourishing in India. Five-star hospitals and private consultants advertise their offers widely to attract rich foreign clients. The advertiser's major interest is to make fast dollars with little concern for the poor people. This type of alarming trend among the present generation of Medical doctors, is not only unsafe to the health of the country and its poor people, but also shows the irresponsibility of the doctors to their professional obligations and welfare of the society.

When I was graduated in medicine, and became a resident doctor, our teachers were primarily academicians. They made thorough research on the natural history of diseases peculiar to India, and published their findings in reputed journals, which were remained as classics in Indian medical literature. When they used to organize medical conferences, they prefer to choose medical colleges as venues, and provided rich scientific content for the intellect. In those days, we used to have economical and simple working lunches. Postgraduate students and junior teachers could easily afford the registration fee for these conferences. A knowledgeable and respected teacher used to inaugurate the conference. The presence of pharmaceutical companies and manufacturers of medical instruments was confined to the exhibition hall, where they display their products in modest stalls. They are not allowed to intrude into the affairs of the conference.

However, in recent times, the trend is changed and almost all the conferences are being organized in seven star hotels, with cocktails and lavish meals. Delegates cannot escape the all-pervading presence of companies selling drugs and medical instruments. Slides on advertising products are projected between two successive talks. We are constantly being told which company has sponsored breakfast, lunch or dinner. At one meeting, the cakes served at tea were embossed with the brand name of the medicines being sold by the company. Senior consultants and their families used to travel by air and lodged in star hotels by pharmaceutical companies. They have chauffeured cars at their disposal all the time. An interesting matter about the conferences is that the dining halls are crowded all the time, but the lecture halls show a progressively diminishing attendance as we proceed from the inauguration of the conference to the last session. The inauguration is performed by a powerful minister in the Government, which is often delayed till the 'dignitary' arrives, by wasting the precious time of thousands of doctors. The press coverage comes in headlines whatever the minister reads from the speech prepared by someone, whereas the research finding presented by the doctors never get due coverage in the news papers.

Thus, there has been a dramatic shift in the value system of medical profession. The commercial relations between some senior members of the profession and the manufacturers of drugs have gone to the extent of neglecting the welfare of the patients. Deliberate demands by doctors for air tickets for themselves and their families, accommodation in five star hotels, and other facilities are linked to promote the interests of drug manufactures. Pharmaceutical companies bring pressure on the doctors who have a huge practice, or a person heading a large institution who can order for goods worth of millions of rupees, or who holds a crucial position in a national medical association, to place orders even for poor quality instruments and drugs. All these immoral practices finally fall on the expenses of the patients who will pay higher prices. The medical council of India, the highest regulatory body in the country, which is supposed to look after the functioning of medical profession on ethical grounds is unfortunately, buried itself up to the neck in the dirt of corruption. Under these circumstances, only God has to save the poor patients, and the tarnished image of the medical profession.

Many hospitals are without clean toilets, freshly laundered bed sheets, pillow covers, and blankets, but the hospital superintendents cheerfully spend huge money on the latest Computerized Tomographic Scanner or Magnetic Resonance Imaging machine for the sake of getting kickbacks from the suppliers. Private hospitals purchase equipment costing millions of U. S. dollars. When the returns do not match the huge capital expenditure, stress is exerted on clinicians and a large number of patients, irrespective of indications for such treatment are referred to the tests, and in turn the doctors receive incentives in the form of mega gifts such as Air conditioners, Refrigerators, Cars etc., Due to such type of immoral practices, the value system of medical profession appears to be degrading day by day. Unfortunately, in the medical curriculum either in the undergraduate or in the postgraduate level there is no course on medical ethics, which is very much needed in the context of present trends in medical practice. The Medical Council of India or the medical education planners should initiate a course in the syllabus of medicine for the students studying medicine.

The medical profession has been constantly changing form the era of Hippocrates to the contemporary times. At one time, it was regarded as a highly divine profession, and the doctor was treated as a

God or equal to God. Thus, there was a popular saying in India, "*vaidyo- narayano- hari*" (the doctor is equal to God), and that glory of the past has lost its relevance today. The bygone days of the physician examining the patient has now turned into "patient examining the doctor", to know whether the doctor is genuine or not, whether he has dedication and care to the patient or money minded. If the medical profession ceases to be noble, and fails to observe the code of conduct prescribed to the doctors, then it must be treated with vigilance and at times with contempt.

In the past the doctors have more concern for their patients, used to study the disease in detail, and suggest the necessary investigations or therapy after considering the financial status of the patient. For this reason, the patients used to have utmost confidence and faith on the doctor, and have great respect to their advice. Patient's faith and confidence on doctors used to cure more ailments than the wonders of the medicine. In recent times, the patients are looking at the doctor with serious doubts. In other words, a patient is examining his doctor whether he is trust worthy, qualified and competent enough to relieve his suffering. This type of a new trend emerged among the patients as a result of increasing corruption in the medical profession. The past glory and sanctity of the medical profession have been buried due to certain evil practices that entered into the medical profession at all levels.

How to Regain the Past Glory?

As already said above, for centuries together, the public treated doctors as Gods. Since four or five decades, the holiness of the doctors has fallen drastically in India due to declining values among doctors in particular and medical practice in general. Currently, only few doctors are regarded as Gods and the rest are treated as devils. If the present trend goes like this, the doctors as well as medical profession become more mechanical, rather than humanistic in the next fifty years

One of the reasons for decline of standards in the medical profession may be due to the failure of the people to identify the right medical personnel, for right medical care, in right time, and it requires some knowledge or consultation of right persons about health care. Some unethical and greedy doctors, irrespective of their competence or specialization, are treating patients suffering from all types of diseases, even though they are not competent to treat those diseases. They never bother to refer such patients to a specialist doctor in that area because they lose their income.

Keeping in mind the present trends of doctors, a stalwart in medical profession Dr. B.C. Roy said: "If you are ill, go to a doctor, take his consultation, and pay him the fees, because doctor must live. Then go to a chemist, buy the medicines, because the chemist must also live. After buying the medicines, throw them in the gutter, because you too must live."

A doctor must remain as a student throughout his life learning new things in his profession. That should be the moral spirit of the doctor, and he must prepare to take that burden if he decides to serve the sick and the disabled with his knowledge and skills. But, how many doctors are updating their knowledge and skills, to save the lives of the patients with dedication and sincerity. The great ancient Indian physician, Charaka rightly said: "Medical men should hold discussions with other medical men. Discussions increase the zeal for knowledge, remove doubts, and strengthen the convictions." It is true, and the spirit behind all the medical conferences is nothing but following the advice of Charka. Medicine and medical practitioners exist to cure diseases to the maximum possible extent, relieve symptoms to the extent enabled by their talents and expertise, and comfort patients at all times.

In the year 1948, the WHO defined health as: "Health Is a State of Complete Physical, Mental, Social, and Spiritual Wellbeing, and not merely an absence of Disease or Infirmity." Therefore, the health professionals engaged in the medical profession should try to satisfy the spirit of this definition by all means. A doctor is not merely someone who diagnosis and prescribes drugs, but also act as a friend, philosopher, and guide to his patients in suggesting solutions to their social, economic, psychological, physical and moral problems. A doctor's pleasing and skillful approach to his patients works more powerful than the use of drugs.

When treating the patient the doctor should not forget that he is treating a human person as a 'whole'. Hence due attention must be paid to his financial, social, psychological and family problems, which are associated with the sickness of a person. In illness there is a plea for love and sympathy, and the doctor has to comfort the patient by his words, expressions, and expertise. Taking appropriate history, frank discussion, sympathetic listening, and thorough physical examinations — are all important facets for correct and in-depth diagnosis of the illness." Sir William Osler aptly says: "it is more important to know what sort of patient has a disease, rather than what sort of disease a patient has."

If the doctors fail to practice the principles of medical ethics, and art of professional knowledge and expertise in the treatment of patients, then they will be held responsible for their negligence and failure. The following Sanskrit couplet, *"Yamarajam Harathu Praanaani, Vaidyarajam Dhanaani Praananeeyu,."* which means: "Yamaraja (the God of death) takes only the life of a person, where as Vaidyaraja (the doctor) takes both the life and wealth of the person he treats. In other words, the Sanskrit couplet describes a careless, greedy, and irresponsible doctor is worse than the Yama, who is known as the God of death by the Hindus.

Unless the community as a whole is vigilant, and takes care of the health care of its people, the days ahead are gloomy, because many fake drugs and false doctors are coming up, destroying the principles of medical ethics, tarnishing the image of medical profession, and disregarding government's health policy.

The principles and practice of medical ethics should be one of the cornerstones of medical education. Mere preaching of ethical values does not make much sense. Teachers and senior medical practitioners must stand as role model for dedication, care, and selfless treatment of patients. The patient should be the centre of attention, and every act being performed keeping in mind his/her welfare. As the cost of medical treatment has gone up, and there is widespread poverty among the people, all efforts must be directed towards providing the best medical care at the least expenses.

As human civilization is steadily progressing, and human morality is evolving to higher and more rational form, let us hope for an ideal health care system, in the years to come, wherein the entire humanity can live with good health, perfect peace, and immense prosperity.

References:

1. Siegerist Henry, *"A History of Medicine"*, Vol. I, (London, Oxford University Press, 1951).

2. Dubos, R.J, *"Man, Medicine and Environment"*, (New York, New American Library, 1969).

3. Nalini Sahay, *"HIV/AIDS counseling:Diagnosis and Management"* in "HIV/AIDS – A Clinicians Perspective," (New Delhi, BI Publications, 2006) pp. 376–377.

4. Lynette Lee Corporal: BALI, Aug 11 2009 (TerraViva/IPS) http://ipsterraviva.asia/2009/08/11/media-missing-the-hivaids-story/

5. Paul A. Volberding, Merle A. Sande, Jocp Lange, Warner C. Greene and Theo Sowa, (eds) *"The Growing problem of AIDS Orphans"* in "Global HIV/AIDS Medicine," Vol. 3, (Philadelphia, Elsevier, 2009), p. 788.

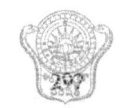

6. Y.V.Satyanarayana, *"Ethics: Theory and Practice"*, (Delhi, Pearson, 2010), p.183.

7. Theo Sowa, *"The Growing Problem of AIDS Orphans"* in Paul A. Volberding, Merle A. Sande, Joep Lange, and Warucr C. Greene, (eds) – "Global HIV/AIDS Medicine", Vol.3, (Philadelphia, Elsevier, 2009), p.788.

8. Dr. Ashwani Bhardwaj, *"AIDS Causes, Prevention and Cure"* (New Delhi, Goodwill Publishing House, 2008), pp.317-329.

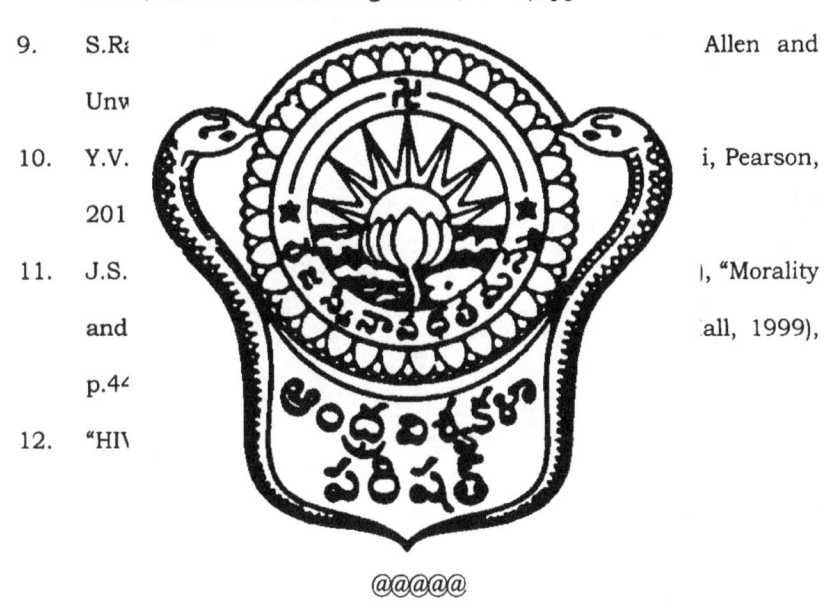

9. S.R٠   Allen and Unv

10. Y.V.   i, Pearson, 201

11. J.S.   ), "Morality and   all, 1999), p.4٠

12. "HI\

CPSIA information can be obtained
at www.ICGtesting.com
Printed in the USA
BVHW071505120123
656165BV00015B/421